A SIMPLER'S GARLAND

THE GENTLE ART OF POULTICING
AND OTHER HERBAL WRITINGS

of
MARINA BOKELMAN

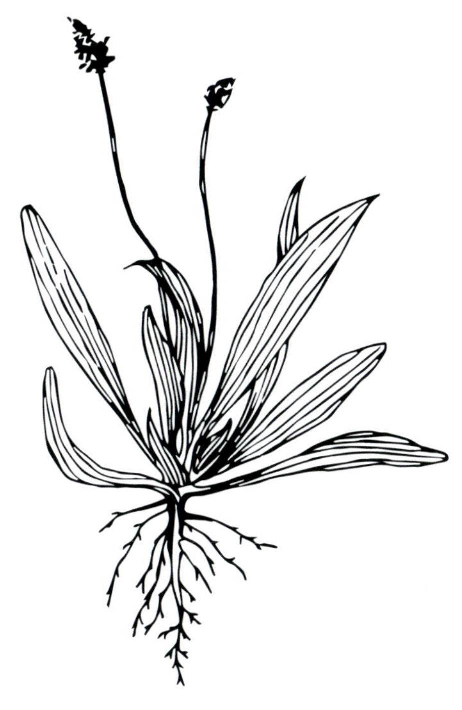

SACRED PAW

2021© All rights reserved

FOR RICK

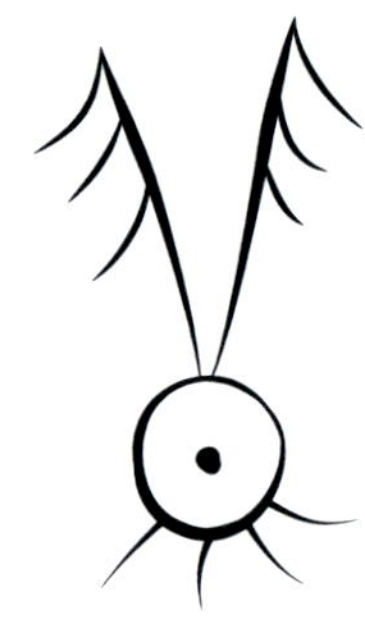

ISBN 979-8-986066-1-8

Pen & Ink plantain illustration by Jacquie Bellon. Line art drawings are stock photos unless otherwise indicated. Book Design & Printing by Jennifer Schrader, Real Graphic

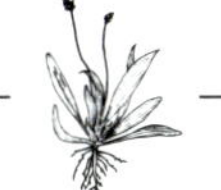

TABLE OF CONTENTS

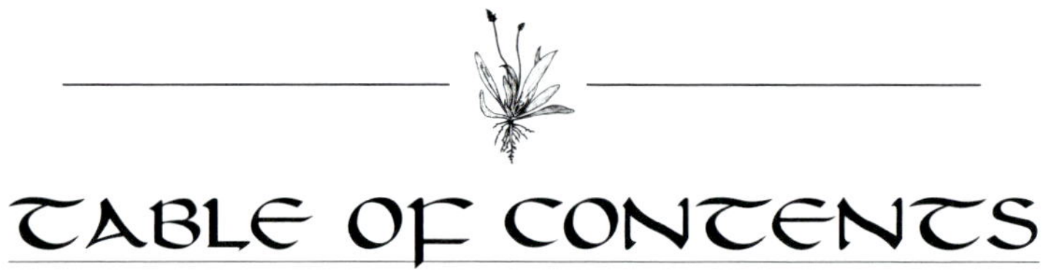

TABLE OF CONTENTS

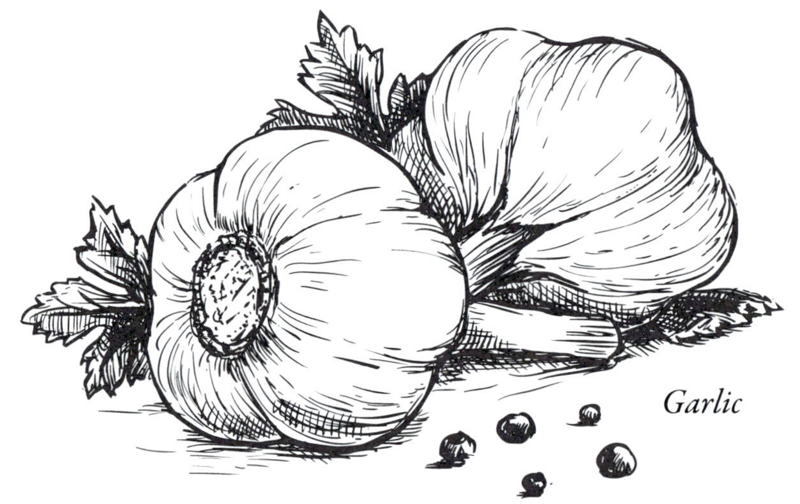

Garlic

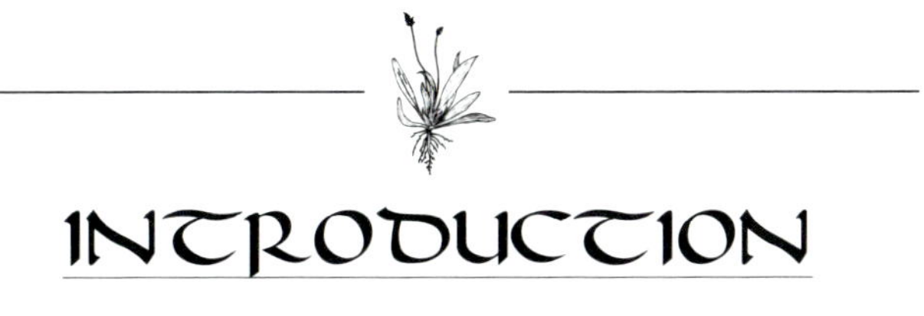

INTRODUCTION

The information provided in these writings is not intended to diagnose or prescribe for any health condition. The information herein is offered as a sharing of personal experiences and anecdotal information. No medical claims are made. Consult a health care professional concerning health problems or conditions. Self-education is the first step toward taking responsibility for healing our bodies and our lives.

Seek out additional information about the herbs mentioned here. Use common sense and trust your intuition. Learn by using herbal remedies on yourself first, then your family, pets and other loved ones. Observe closely and remember what you learn. Take notes. Once you have had success, you will never forget the herb or the protocol. In this way your knowledge, confidence in yourself and trust in the herbs will grow.

Remember, you do not need to learn all the herbs—over time you will develop a special relationship with a handful of healing plants and your own favorite protocols for using them. Learn the common herbs, especially the ones that are common in your habitat. They are often the most useful and are certainly the most accessible. Don't forget that culinary herbs have medicinal properties. Culinary herbs are easy to grow in your garden or in a flower pot. And you can buy organic culinary herbs at a health food store or co-op. Simple remedies are often the best.

Look for herbals written by experienced clinical herbalists because they write about what they themselves know from personal experience. You quickly learn to discern which books were written by people with direct experience.

My first go-to books are *Herbal Handbook for Everyone* by Juliette de Bairacli-Levy, and *A Modern Herbal in two volumes* by Maud Grieve. I just came back from a quick trip to the bookshelf with an armful of books I have found to be useful at various stages of my life with herbs and herbal medicine. Each offers something different, original, and eminently useful. In no particular order:

- *The Herb Book* by John Lust
- *Medicinal Plants of the Mountain West* by Michael Moore
- *Health Secrets of Plants and Herbs* by Maurice Messegue
- *Nature's Healing Agents* by R. Swinburne Clymer, M.D.
- *Herbal Healing for Women* by Rosemary Gladstar
- *Back to Eden* by Jethro Kloss
- *The Roots of Health* by Leon Petulengro
- *Heal Yourself with Vegetables, Fruits and Grains* by Jean Valnet, M.D.

A *Simpler* is an herbalist who uses simple remedies, often using a single herb. In the olden days these remedies were called "simples", and this particular way of working with herbs was called "simpling", or "granny medicine". A *Garland* is an archaic term referring to a pamphlet or small book of short pieces, usually relating to a single subject.

As a Simpler of herbs, this Garland of writings is my offering to you.

May All Beings Benefit

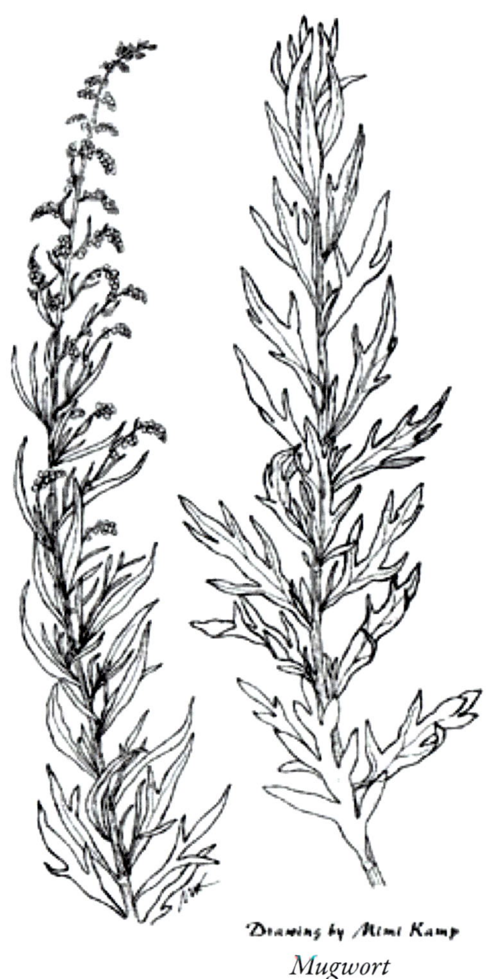

Drawing by Mimi Kamp

Mugwort

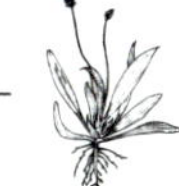

POULTICES AND RELATED PROTOCOLS

THE GENTLE ART OF POULTICING

A mosquito bites you while you are working in your garden—put a *plantain* poultice on it. Your husband sprains his ankle playing volleyball—put a compound *mullein* poultice on it. Your child has a chest cold—put an *onion* poultice on it.

A poultice is a method of applying herbs directly to the skin, usually employing moist heat. It is one of the oldest and most basic of all herbal remedies. The first poultice was undoubtedly a pad of soothing green leaves chewed and applied to the injury. Poultices remain a basic and satisfying item in the home remedy repertoire. Perhaps this is because making and applying a poultice is such a direct expression of the healing touch itself.

Why Use a Poultice

When a poultice is applied to an injury immediately after it happens, I have found that almost all the typical pain, swelling, inflammation and other complications can be prevented. In general, herbal poultices are used to
- ~ draw out toxins,
- ~ soothe and relieve pain,
- ~ reduce swelling and inflammation,
- ~ increase local circulation,
- ~ promote healing of sores, wounds and traumatic injuries,
- ~ dissolve small cysts and tumors.

How to Apply a Poultice

Because a poultice is a moist, pulpy or pasty affair, it is usually spread on a clean cotton cloth (warmed in advance if you wish) and bound over the skin, poultice side down. If especially gloppy, the herbal mass can be sandwiched between two pieces of sturdy cheesecloth. The poultice may then be bound in place with another clean dry cloth. Change as needed, depending on the ailment or the type of poultice used. A *mustard* plaster, which is made with a *very hot herb*, must always be applied between two nice, smooth cotton cloths, NOT cheesecloth. Apply the plaster two to four times a day, depending on the severity of the condition, and only for a few minutes at a time—just until the skin begins to turn pink. Remove the plaster promptly as there is a real danger of burning the skin. A soothing *comfrey* poultice on the other hand would be changed every hour, or half hour until relief is obtained. With a drawing poultice the rule of thumb is to change it when the herbs become warm—this means they have drawn heat out of the injury and should be changed to continue to draw off the inflammation.

Regarding Cheesecloth:

Your best source of cheesecloth is a fabric or craft supply store. Supermarket cheesecloth is so flimsy it is useless. However if that is all you can get, use 2-4 layers to sandwich your poultice.

POULTICE MATERIALS

Raw Green Herbs

The simplest poultice is made of fresh, green herbs, either chewed or pounded into a pulpy mass in a wooden bowl with a wooden pestle. Chewing an herb and applying it to a wound or other injury may seem repellent to some people, but Native American and other folk medical practices around the world document this as a common practice. My mother, a registered nurse, taught me that the *saliva* of a healthy person is mildly antiseptic and that licking or sucking a wound is an instinctive act based on sound principles. As an anthropological side note, the *saliva* of a healthy dog is highly antiseptic, and in some cultures a dog would be invited to lick the wound—perhaps you have heard the expression "clean as a hound's tooth" which refers to this property of canine *saliva.*

Plantain is the herb most often used as a chewed poultice, most specifically for the bites of mosquitos and other stinging insects. Since *plantain* is so abundant in lawns, gardens and waste acres, it is hard to imagine being out of reach of this simple folk remedy. Simply wash or dust off the leaf, chew into a bolus and apply to the injury. Both broad and narrow leaf *plantain* are equally valuable.

Virtually any chlorophyll-rich, **non-poisonous** plant leaves may be used for a poultice. The most common and beneficial are *comfrey, mallow, plantain, dock, mullein, cabbage, sorrel* and *violet leaves,* which are especially cooling and mucilaginous. These plants are common and may be identified with the help of any good plant identification book or a botanical friend. They may also be grown in your garden. Any salad green may be added to your list of poultice plants, including *iceberg lettuce.* I think it is comforting to know that the vegetable drawer of your refrigerator can supply you with poultice materials, even if you are not a wilderness wildcrafter or avid herb gardener.

My favorite method is to pound the chosen leaves in a wooden bowl with a wooden pestle.

Keep pounding and turning the leaves until a moist, pulpy mass is achieved, but well before you liquefy the plant material. This pounding, like chewing, breaks down the tough cellulose cell walls of the plant and releases healing juices. Next, take a double layer of cheesecloth and spread the poultice material on half of it. Fold over the unused half, place over the injured part and bind in place with a clean cloth. I find that dampening the binding cloth with *natural apple cider vinegar* speeds absorption of the healing properties of the herbs. The *apple cider vinegar* further softens the plant cellulose and seems also to increase permeability of the skin. Lacking cheese cloth, I have often simply placed the moist, pulpy plant material directly on my skin and bound it on with whatever clean cloth was available, or held it on with my hand for first aid relief.

This type of poultice is applied at room temperature and should be changed as soon as it becomes warm. You will be surprised at how effectively these fresh herbal poultices absorb the heat generated by inflammation or traumatic injury such as sprain or contusion. Experience will teach you how to tell the difference between the warmth of ordinary body temperature and the extra heat the poultice absorbs from the injury.

I once used a simple *comfrey* poultice of pounded fresh leaves wrapped with an *apple cider vinegar-*soaked cloth when I was thrown from a big horse onto a hard gravel bank, badly spraining my arm and shoulder. The relief after each fresh application of *comfrey* was remarkable. And there was no bruising!

Another method of using raw green herbs is to gently heat the leaves in a small amount of water until they become soft and supple. This is especially effective with tough leaves such as *cabbage. Mullein* leaves may be rinsed and then soaked in *hot apple cider vinegar* to soften and activate. The hairy leaves of mullein are often dusty and the prickles can be uncomfortable unless the leaves are softened first. Place softened leaves between layers of cheesecloth, or if the leaves are large and have sufficient body, bind them directly onto the skin with a clean cloth.

Raw Roots

Certain roots, such as *carrot, parsnip*, and *horseradish*, have great virtue as poultice plants. These plants should be grated, placed between layers of doubled cheesecloth (retaining the juice as much as you can) and bound onto the affected part with a clean, dry or *apple cider vinegar* dampened cloth. Roots have tremendous power to draw, and are especially useful for boils, abscesses, cysts, pus-filled wounds and tumors. *Horseradish* is a *very hot herb*. Prepare as for a *mustard* plaster and diligently monitor the skin beneath the poultice, removing it as soon as the skin barely begins to show pink.

Raw Garlic

Raw *garlic* is in a category all by itself. It is an unparalleled drawing agent, as well as being strongly antiseptic. It was once jokingly referred to as "Russian penicillin" for its antibiotic properties. If there is need, you can place raw *garlic* pulp directly onto a festering sore to cleanse it. Apply *olive oil* around the sore to prevent the *garlic* from affecting the surrounding area. *Garlic* is a *hot herb* and will cause a strong burning sensation but it will do no harm.

Raw *garlic*, taken internally, will cleanse the bloodstream in four minutes. This is why you can eat raw *garlic* and soon thereafter detect an odor on the breath. The cleansing properties of *garlic* have travelled through the bloodstream to be excreted by the lungs along with it all the toxins it has absorbed. It is the toxins that are smelled on the breath, not the *garlic* itself. When I worked in the library at the University of North Carolina in Cullowhee I ate two raw cloves of *garlic* every morning on an empty stomach. Never once, in this very public setting, did anyone detect *garlic* on my breath. This was because I was healthy and living clean—raising all my food myself and using herbs for my medicine.

For seven years I had my *Medicine Flower* Herbal Remedies booth at the Northern California Renaissance Faire near Novato. For the six weeks of the Faire I was the village herbalist. Faire folk came to me with their problems, during the day and after hours as well.

One evening a vendor came to my booth with an abscessed tooth—his cheek was swollen as if he had a golf ball tucked into it. He was in terrible pain and would not be able to get to a dentist until the following Tuesday (it was Saturday).

I advised him to peel a clove of raw *garlic* and place it into his cheek next to the abscessed tooth. I asked him to be careful not to nick it because the *garlic* juice would produce an unpleasant (though harmless) burning sensation to the mucus membranes of his mouth. I asked him to change it for a fresh clove every half hour as the *garlic* would quickly become saturated with toxins and by-products of inflammation. I suggested he eat one to two cloves of *garlic*, cut in tiny pieces and swallowed with water every hour at first, and then every two to three hours thereafter. I suggested he follow this protocol for 24 hours.

He came to my booth the next day with a smile on his face and a perfectly flat cheek. He had followed the protocol faithfully through the night. He said at the 24th hour the pain had turned off "like a lightbulb". This greatly increased the esteem I already had for *garlic*!

I always use raw *garlic* internally to speed the healing of any condition where there is inflammation, infection or toxicity. I also use it preventatively.

Cucurbits

Although neither roots nor green herbs, members of the squash family, the *cucurbitaceae*, provide useful poulticing material with a broad spectrum of actions, from drawing to cooling. Slices of *pumpkin*, roasted and applied as hot as can be tolerated, are wonderful to draw boils and other similar afflictions. Peeled slices of *cucumber* are cooling and famous for providing relief to tired, puffy eyes. Use *cucumber* whenever a cooling and soothing effect is desired. I would not hesitate to grate *zucchini* and use it as a poultice.

Dried Herbs

In order to be used in a poultice, dried herbs must be mixed with some kind of carrying and thickening agent. These compound poultices often require some cooking to achieve the required thick paste which is then spread hot onto a clean, dry cloth (pre-heated if you wish) and bound, poultice side down, over the injured or aching part. Even a single layer of high quality cheesecloth on top of the paste will keep it from messily glopping off as you apply it.

The most commonly used thickening agents are *bran, powdered oats, powdered flax seeds* and *slippery elm bark powder*. These plant materials have soothing and healing properties of their own which are enhanced by the addition of the specifically medicinal herbs. *Oat flakes* and *flax seeds* may be whirled in a blender to make a coarse powder or used whole, which requires more cooking.

The rule of thumb is to mix equal parts of the dried herb and the thickening agent and then vigorously stir in enough hot water to make a thick paste. If you have nothing else in the house, *wheat bread* (crust removed) soaked in *hot milk* or water, or *tofu* (squeezed free of excess moisture) may be used as a poultice base.

These compound poultices are more versatile in the type of treatment you can accomplish. For an infected wound, antiseptic herbs such as *yarrow, rosemary, wormwood* and *thyme* can be used. In cases of stiffness, penetrating and heating herbs such as *rosemary* and *cayenne* (the latter used sparingly) might be added to your formula. For aches and pains, anodynes such as *hops* and *chamomile* would be the herbs of choice. For a sprain, *mullein* (which reduces swelling and relieves pain) may be combined with *lobelia* (an anti-spasmodic) and *cayenne* (which creates heat and increases local circulation) to create a rather sophisticated treatment. Consult several good herbal reference books and make your choice of herbs based on the effect you desire. Always use common sense when compounding. When trying a new herb, err on the side of caution.

Powdered Herbs

Golden Seal and **Myrrh** are two powerful antiseptic herbs which I always have on hand in case of emergencies. *Myrrh* is also astringent, making it useful when there is bleeding.

More than once I have sprinkled the combination of these two herbs directly into a fresh, open wound. On one occasion the hatchet I was using to chop kindling slipped and cut the side of the first knuckle (the one nearest the hand) of my forefinger to the bone. I filled the wound with the two powders and taped a pad of clean cloth over it, applying pressure until the bleeding very quickly stopped. The wound healed swiftly, and there was no infection or complication of any kind.

Rosemary and **Wormwood**, in equal quantities, finely powdered and then rubbed through a sieve, are a superlative antiseptic and healing combination. I have used *rosemary* and *wormwood* powder with near miraculous results.

The first occasion was when a newly sharpened kitchen knife surprised me with a long cut deep into the soft flesh near the fingertip of my forefinger. This was a deep, scary, gaping wound which would normally have required at least five stitches. However, I was living deep in the Smoky Mountains with the nearest hospital two hours away and besides, I was a young herbalist and this was a golden opportunity. I filled the wound with the combination of *rosemary* and *wormwood* powder, fashioned a couple of butterfly bandages out of tape to hold the lips of the wound together, quickly bound it up with a nice clean rag, and applied pressure until the bleeding very quickly abated. I made a very strong tea of the two herbs and frequently wet the binding cloth with the brew. I did not unwrap the dressing for over a week because I didn't want to disturb the healing process, and because I was a little scared to look at it. There was no pain, itching or inflammation, and healing was speedy. For a little while the finger was stiff and also numb from nerves having been cut. But the numbness went away in time. A thin white line of scar tissue is all I have to remind me of my adventure.

Here is another example. When I lived in the mountains of North Carolina I had a big flock of free living Banty-Game chickens that roosted in the plum tree outside my kitchen door. One evening I noticed that one of my little hens was not able to fly up into the tree. When I picked her up I discovered that she had been struck by a hawk. There were deep rips and gouges in her shoulder muscles and at the base of her neck where she had been struck with the hawk's talons, and her back was completely naked and raw. It was clear that as she ran forward to escape the clutches of the hawk, the skin had been peeled off her back as neatly as if she had been skinned.

I immediately put her in an orange crate in the living room. I coated her back thickly with the combination *rosemary* and *wormwood* powder, completely filling the deep gouges in her shoulder muscles. I then very carefully wet the powder on her back and neck with a strong infusion of the

two herbs. I placed a nice clean rag soaked with the herbal brew over her back. I made sure the rag was wet with the herb tea all day, every day.

After one week I cautiously lifted the rag and saw new skin with pin feathers beginning to sprout up through the herb crust! After two weeks I let her out of the crate and she ran around the living room exercising her wings. On the third week I let her outside and she flew back into the tree. As you can imagine, this greatly strengthened my faith in the healing power of these two herbs!

N.B. Herbs to be used in this way for open wound treatment must be finely powdered and of the highest quality, organically grown for preference. Whirl in a blender if you have one or pound thoroughly with a mortar and pestle, then rub through a sieve. Store in a glass container and keep away from light, heat and moisture.

A FEW POULTICE RECIPES

Flaxseed Poultice
This is a classic recipe. Sprinkle 4 ounces of ground *flaxseed* into 1 pint of boiling water, stirring vigorously. Add 1 Tb *olive oil*. Spread on a warm cloth and apply. *Flaxseed* by itself is soothing and drawing. Depending on the desired effect you can add other herbs, grated fresh or dried.

Onion Poultice
This is another classic. Chop 2 medium *onions* and sauté very lightly in *olive oil*. Add 1 cup powdered *oat flakes* and sufficient boiling water to make a thick mush. Cook for a few minutes. This is a gentle but effective decongestant poultice for the lungs. You may add *essential oil of eucalyptus* (from a few drops to 1 tsp, depending on your tolerance and the quality of the oil) for extra

penetrating and disinfecting qualities. *Eucalyptus* has an affinity for the lungs. This was the go-to remedy for pneumonia in the days before antibiotics. *Garlic* and other antiseptic and decongestant herbs should be taken internally and the poultice changed at regular intervals. I would not hesitate to use this treatment for pneumonia if there was no alternative. In addition, I would fast the patient on *honey* and *lemon juice* and administer raw *garlic* for internal disinfection. Remember—when you use an herbal remedy for a serious condition, you must make a whole-hearted commitment to the treatment and follow through. No half-hearted measures!

Compound Mullein Poultice
Mix together 3 parts *slippery elm bark* powder, 2 parts *mullein* (crushed or powdered), 1 part

lobelia (crushed or powdered) and 1/4 to 1/3 part *cayenne pepper*. Stir in enough hot water to make a paste. This would be especially helpful for the swelling, stiffness and pain of a sprain or strain. The cayenne will create a heating effect. Watch out for reddening of the skin.

Mustard Plaster

Another classic. Mix together ½ cup powdered *yellow mustard seed* and ½ cup *whole wheat flour*. Stir in hot water to make a paste. Add 1 Tb *apple cider vinegar*. For children and others with sensitive skin, add 1 *raw egg white*. **CAUTION: *Mustard* plasters should be applied between two cotton cloths (*not* cheesecloth), NEVER directly to the skin.** Sit by the side of the patient and check the skin under the poultice cloth *frequently*. When the skin begins to show signs of

pink, remove the plaster immediately. Apply twice a day. *Mustard* plasters can be applied alternately to chest and back for pulmonary congestion, or over the kidney area in cases of kidney inflammation. It is deeply penetrating, antiseptic and *very hot*. **Please be careful with this one.**

Clay

Although not an herb, *clay* belongs in everyone's medicine cabinet. It has great drawing powers. Different clays have different properties—*green clay* is different from *bentonite*. A discussion of *clay* is beyond the scope of this writing. If you can find it, *Our Earth, Our Cure* by Raymond Dextreit, translated and edited by Michel Abehsera, has an excellent discussion of how to use *clay* internally and externally.

COMMON SENSE CAUTIONS

In general, do not attempt home treatment without the advice of a trusted health care provider. In particular, ***do not treat pain, stiffness or swelling of the abdomen without diagnosis***. It may be an appendix or a pair of ovaries on the way to rupturing.

If you are gathering your own herbs, be certain of your identification before using any plant. Not every broad leaved green plant is your friend. Do not gather medicinal plants closer than 100 feet from the road as they will be saturated with exhaust emissions.

Go slowly when trying a new herb—everyone is allergic to something. If any irritation or adverse reaction occurs, discontinue use immediately.

Self-education is the key. Even among the medicinal plants in your herb book, many are not appropriate for making poultices. And some, like *Poke* (*Phytolacca americana*) which are supremely useful in the hands of a skilled practitioner for specific conditions, may be deadly.

POULTICE HERBS AND THEIR PROPERTIES

Choose your poultice herbs based on their properties and the result you wish to obtain. Do you need to disinfect, draw out toxins, soothe and relax, promote new tissue growth, reduce swelling, relieve congestion, or relax muscle spasms? All herbs have multiple virtues—choose the ones that will give you the

most for the given situation. You might choose antiseptic herbs for treating new wounds. If a wound becomes inflamed or festers, you may wish to add herbs with the ability to draw toxins. At the same time you may wish to soothe the inflamed tissues with cooling and demulcent herbs.

There are times where I will make reference to the *Standard Brew*, which is one of Juliette de Bairacli-Levy's methods of preparing an herbal infusion. Here is how to prepare the *Standard Brew*. Put 1 large handful of dried herbs into 2 cups of cold water in a glass, stainless steel or unchipped enamel vessel. Gently bring to a simmer (do *not* boil) and hold at that heat for 3 minutes, keeping the vessel covered to avoid losing delicate healing properties. Remove from heat and steep with herbs in the brew for at least 5-30 minutes— overnight is best. You can leave herbs in the Brew and store, covered, in the fridge. Roots, being harder, need to be gently boiled until softened. You will find what works for you.

Bran (*Triticum* species) is tonic and soothing for skin afflictions. It is a time-honored carrying agent for compound herbal poultices and has drawing properties of its own. It is especially effective applied warm or hot.

Cabbage (*Brassica oleracea*) is strongly absorptive of toxins and the by-products of infection, hence useful for wounds, infections, skin ulcers, skin eruptions and other inflamed conditions. Remove the tough central ribs and crush the *cabbage* leaves gently with a rolling pin or blanch with boiling water. Alternatively, heat slowly and simmer gently in a small amount of water until the leaves are semi-translucent and supple. This is the method I have used the most. Another method of preparing *cabbage* leaves is to macerate them in warm *olive oil* for an additional soothing action.

Cabbage is so powerful it may cause a temporary flare-up or healing crisis especially in long standing chronic conditions. Suspend use, and soothe with warm *olive oil*, or switch to poultices of *lettuce* or *comfrey*. Then continue with more moderate applications, or alternate *cabbage* with *lettuce*.

Carrot (*Daucus carota*) is tonic and drawing in its action. Scrub well, peel if necessary, and grate finely, retaining all the juice. The high Vitamin A content helps speed healing.

Cayenne (*Capsicum annuum, C. frutescens*) is one of the most powerful and safest stimulants in the

herbal kingdom. It is also a powerful disinfectant. It is rubefacient, warming and increases local circulation, making it a useful ingredient in compound poultices for stiff, sore muscles and joints. Use sparingly in combination with other herbs, at the rate of no more than 1/16 to 1/8 parts *cayenne* in the total formula. Start with the least amount and increase gradually as you note the effects. The strength of *cayenne* varies greatly. Some herb companies list different BTUs (heat units) for the *capsicums* they sell. Learn what works best for you so that you do not cause over-stimulation or discomfort beyond your tolerance level.

Chamomile (*Anthemis nobilis*) is an anodyne and mild anti-spasmodic, also very soothing and gently cleansing to the skin.

Comfrey (*Symphytum officinale*) should be in everyone's poultice repertoire. It contains *allantoin* which promotes cellular regeneration, making it a powerful aid for the healing of bruises, swellings, sprains and strains of muscles, tendons, and ligaments. It is anti-inflammatory, analgesic, and astringent.

The fresh root, which is more astringent than the leaves, may be grated or pulped and used as a hot or cold application. Like other astringent herbs it is useful for treating wounds and stopping bleeding. The pulped fresh root is also *extremely mucilaginous* to the point of feeling slimy if pounded too much. (If this ever happens to you, just smear it all over your body as a marvelous healing moisturizer). Taken internally as a tea, *comfrey* speeds healing of all injuries, including broken bones as its folk name "knitbone" attests. *Comfrey* contains *silica*, which the body is able to transmute into calcium—this accounts for its ability to speed the knitting of broken bones. **Cleavers** (*Galium aparine*), aka *Goosegrass* or *Bedstraw* also contains silica. Of the silicaceous herbs **Horsetail** (*Equisetum arvense*) is the richest by far. You must be careful with the internal use of *horsetail* as the high silica content which is responsible for its healing power can also irritate the kidneys. Dosage is in the realm of 2 Tb of the *Standard Brew* several times a day.

<u>*Dock*</u> (*Rumex crispus*) makes a cooling and drawing poultice useful for inflammation, rashes, sores, skin eruptions and engorged breasts.

<u>*Flax Seed*</u> (*Linum usitatissimum*), when ground and used in a poultice, is emollient, demulcent and promotes drainage and healing of wounds, infections, abscesses, boils, swellings, sprains and strains. Note that "usitatissimum" in the Latin binomial means "supremely, superlatively useful".

<u>*Garlic*</u> (*Allium sativum*) shares the same properties as *onions* and is powerful for drawing toxins. It is useful as a topical application for skin parasites like ringworm. *Garlic* can be pulped in a wooden mortar and pestle, smashed with the broad side of a sturdy chef's knife, or simply squeezed through your *garlic* press.

Garlic is a powerfully stimulating and antiseptic *hot herb*—be sure to wash your hands after handling freshly cut, pulped and juicy *garlic. Garlic* will do no harm, but the burning sensation on mucous membranes is very uncomfortable. If applying to a festering sore, smooth *olive oil* on the surrounding skin to prevent possible irritation. Raw *garlic*, taken internally, will speed healing of wounds, sores and the like through its ability to cleanse the bloodstream within four minutes of ingestion.

<u>*Hops*</u> (*Humulus lupulus*) are a useful anodyne and nervine, both internally and externally. *Hops* poultices are useful for wounds, sores, rashes, boils, cysts, swellings, aches and inflammations.

<u>*Horseradish*</u> (*Cochlearia armoracia*) has antibacterial, stimulating and penetrating qualities which make it useful as a poultice for wounds, sores, swellings, tumors, and stiff muscles and joints. This is a *very hot herb*, so apply the grated root between two cotton cloths (not cheese cloth). Please monitor your poultice carefully and remove when skin begins to look slightly pink. Like all *hot herbs*, remove the poultice well before a hot or burning sensation is felt.

<u>*Lettuce*</u> (*Lactuca sativa*) is a mild, soothing poultice material. You can alternate *lettuce* and *cabbage* poultices for an alternation of soothing and

stimulating/drawing effects. It shares, to a much milder degree, the anodyne properties of *Wild Lettuce* (*Lactuca serriola* or *Lactuca virosa*). *Wild Lettuce* is a bit too prickly to use as a direct poultice, but the white juice may be expressed and blended with other materials for relief of pain or used straight to treat warts.

<u>*Lobelia*</u> (*Lobelia inflata*) is noted for its antispasmodic properties. Internally it is used in combination with *cayenne*, which balances its powerful relaxant properties. Combine with *mullein* and other herbs for swellings, sprains, strains and stiff muscles and joints.

<u>*Mallow*</u> (*Malva sylvestris, M. rotundifolia*) is soothing, absorptive and demulcent, thanks to its high mucilage content. Pound or chew the cleaned leaves and apply to sores, wounds, inflammations and skin irritations. If you do not have access to wild *mallow*, you may substitute the leaves of the common garden *hollyhock*, to which it is related. As is often the case, the tame garden cultivar is much less potent than its wild relative.

<u>*Mullein*</u> (*Verbascum thapsus*) is mildly germicidal. Its analgesic properties make it a very useful poultice for swellings, inflammation, sprains and strains. The leaves, soaked in *hot apple cider vinegar*, make a good poultice for swollen glands. *Mullein* has an affinity for dry, disturbed ground, although it was a common cottage garden plant in England.

<u>*Mustard Seed*</u> (*Brassica nigra* or *Sinapsis alba*) is a powerful antiseptic and penetrating irritant. Powdered *mustard seed* is used to make a plaster which increases circulation and breaks up congestion and inflammation of the lungs. It is also useful for pain and stiffness of muscles and joints. **<u>*Never, ever*</u>** apply a *mustard* plaster directly to the skin, always between cotton cloths. Monitor your plaster and remove it promptly when the skin begins to turn slightly pink in order to avoid burning.

<u>*Onion*</u> (*Allium cepa*) is drawing, antiseptic, penetrating, decongestive and absorptive. Useful in pulmonary complaints. An *onion* poultice is the classic treatment for all lung congestions, including pneumonia.

Onion is a powerful absorbant of toxins and waste products. If you save a piece of leftover raw onion in the refrigerator, it will absorb the outgassing from whatever you have wrapped or stored it in, PLUS whatever else is in the stale air inside your refrigerator. I never save an unused piece of *onion* (or *garlic*). By the same token, you could put a bowl of cut *onions* in the sick room where the ailment is infectious! Be sure to change the *onions* frequently. The folk practice of wearing cloves of *garlic* in a cloth pouch around the neck (over the thymus gland which is part of the immune systsem) is based on the ability of the *alliums* to draw toxins to themselves.

Parsnip (*Pastinaca sativa*) is a tonic and drawing root, useful for boils, abscesses and swellings. Grate it as you would *carrots*.

Plantain (*Plantago major, P. lanceolata*) is an important poultice herb for bites, stings, wounds and inflamed conditions. It is cooling, soothing, mucilaginous and mildly astringent. It has the great virtue of being found almost everywhere as a "weed" in lawns and gardens. It is worth disturbing a little piece of ground just to get the medicinal herbs such as *plantain, dock, dandelion, cleavers, mullein* and *shepherd's purse* to grow.

Potato (*Solanum tuberosum*) is soothing and healing when grated and applied to burns and sores. Some *olive oil* may be added. Folk medicine is full of references to raw potato (white or Irish only) as a burn remedy. If there is no time to grate the *potato*, simply slice it open and apply the juicy side to the burn. It also has drawing properties.

Pumpkin (*Cucurbita maxima*) has tremendous drawing powers when applied as hot as can be tolerated to boils and abscesses.

Rosemary (*Rosmarinus officinalis*) is an antiseptic, astringent and penetrating herb, useful alone or in combination for wounds, bites, stings and stiffness. May be pounded fresh or used dried. My favorite antiseptic combination is *rosemary* and *wormwood,* dried and finely powdered in a mortar and pestle or blender and then rubbed through a sieve. I have sprinkled these two herbs directly

into a wound, and bound it with some green leaves (*plantain, lettuce*) and a nice clean rag.

Shepherd's Purse (*Capsella bursa-pastoris) is* one of the smaller *Cruciferae* (aka *Brassicas*). The plant is tiny and the seed pods which give it its name are like plump little inverted hearts filled with golden seeds. *Shepherd's Purse* is antiseptic and strongly astringent. It can be used as a styptic, applied as a direct poultice to staunch bleeding. Use a strong tea to bathe a wound, or apply in the form of a cold compress. I love *Shepherd's Purse* and consider myself lucky if it volunteers in my garden or grows wild in my habitat.

Slippery Elm Bark (*Ulmus fulva*) is a supremely useful demulcent and emollient poultice, absorbing toxins and promoting healing of all irritated, inflamed and ulcerated tissues. The powder is a superb base for a compound poultice. Whether used internally or externally, it heals whatever it touches. Unfortunately, due to irresponsible wildcrafting and Dutch Elm disease, it is very difficult to find a powder of the true inner bark of this valuable medicine tree.

Sorrel (*Rumex acetosa*), also called *Sheep Sorrel* or *Sour Grass*, is a cooling poultice for skin eruptions, sores, abscesses, skin ulcers, tumors and boils. Pulp well and apply cold. It is an old remedy for skin cancers.

Thyme (*Thymus vulgaris, T. serpyllum*) is a powerfully antiseptic and penetrating herb. Like *Rosemary* it stimulates circulation, hastening wound healing. It is useful not only for wounds, but for abscesses and a variety of inflammatory conditions.

Violet (*Viola odorata*) is prized for its cooling, soothing, emollient, demulcent and powerfully dissolvent properties. It is used as a poultice for boils, abscesses, tumors and a variety of other skin afflictions.

___Yarrow___ (*Achillea millefolium*) is named for Achilles, the great warrior healer. He studied healing with Chiron, who also taught Asclepius. Achilles used this plant to poultice the wounds of his soldiers. Yarrow is a strong astringent (helpful to staunch bleeding) and antiseptic— perfect for wounds inflicted by the sharp metal edges of swords. Preferably leaves but also the blossoms may be pounded fresh or used dried in a compound poultice or as a cold compress.

THE POWER OF CABBAGE

One of the most powerful healing herbs is one of the most humble of all vegetables—the *cabbage.*

Cabbage first came to my attention when I read *Heal Yourself with Vegetables, Fruits & Grains* by Jean Valnet, M.D. (Cornerstone Library, NY, 1975, 1976). The entry devoted to *cabbage* ran to 20 pages, while all other entries got a page or two at the most. Maurice Messegue, the noted French herbal healer who got miraculous results through the use of external application *only* (compresses, fomentations, hand and foot baths) also spoke highly of *cabbage* in *Health Secrets of Plants and Herbs*, (William Morrow & Co., NY, 1979).

Therefore, when faced with a truly daunting (and dangerous) situation, that of incipient gangrene, I immediately turned to the *cabbage* poultice.

First I will describe how to make a *cabbage* poultice. You must find a large, beautiful head of *green* cabbage, wash it and peel away any of the outer leaves that are damaged. Now, using a small, very sharp knife carefully incise the tough central midribs of the outermost leaves and gently peel off the freed half leaves which now do not cling so tightly. Once you have a neat stack of the smooth half leaves you can prepare them for use. You will also have

cabbage leaves that are wrinkled and folded in on themselves, but don't worry—you can still use much of it.

My method is to very gently warm the chosen leaves in very little water until they become pliable and slightly translucent. These warm, softened *cabbage* leaves can now be laid three to six layers thick on the wound or condition you are treating. Alternative methods for preparing the leaves after removing the central ribs are to gently crush the leaves with a rolling pin or bottle, or macerate them in warm *olive oil*. Or you can pour boiling water over the leaves and soak until ready for use.

Now I will tell you my first experience with using *cabbage* as a poultice.

In the 1980s my boyfriend, Rick Peltier, was a construction worker. After a concrete pour where he knelt on uncured concrete with levis torn at the knees, he developed septic burns where the unprotected skin of his knees touched the concrete. Uncured concrete is corrosive. After a couple of days, when he finally let me look at his knees, I believed I was looking at incipient gangrene. What had initially looked like a series of small burns had developed into large ugly sores. The inflammation around the puffy margins was a deep, angry red, and the centers had become black and necrotic, shaped like inverted volcanos as the corrosion ate deeper and deeper into the flesh, heading towards the bone. I did not like the look or smell of these sores.

I did not give my boyfriend a choice. I prepared the *cabbage* leaves using the gentle warming in water method as described above, and bound a layer six leaves thick over the affected area. I covered the poultice with a nice clean rag, and bound it in place around each knee with larger rags, finishing off with an Ace bandage to hold all in place.

The very next morning, when I unwrapped his knees, I was met with an astonishing sight. The angry red inflammation had disappeared, leaving a narrow margin of pink. The black, necrotic areas had likewise disappeared, leaving only moist, pink flesh with small islands of granulation—indicating the creation of healthy, new tissue. I continued the treatment for two more days until the sores were healed enough to go to an herbal salve and band-aids.

This experience blew my mind and gave me a deep and abiding faith in the healing power of the *cabbage* poultice. So twenty years later I turned immediately to *cabbage* for healing a serious wound. This experience is described in detail in the section on Compound Poultices.

Most recently, I used a simple *cabbage* poultice for healing a deep, festering burn.

This experience I will briefly describe.

I burned my arm while extending it deeply into a wood stove to tend a fire. The burns delivered by the hot, ashy iron of the wood stove were very deep—they were at least second degree burns. This burn I first treated with my *Elder Sisters Healing Herbal Salve,* which is unparalleled as a powerful antiseptic, analgesic and anti-inflammatory salve. It heals ordinary burns and scalds with only a couple applications. But *Elder Sisters* was powerless before this degree of burn and it began to fester quite painfully. At this point I turned to the simple *cabbage* poultice which I prepared as described above. I applied the warm, damp, pliant leaves four layers thick, covering them with a nice clean rag pad and binding it all on with a bandanna. The next day all pain was gone and after a couple more *cabbage* poultices what had been a terrible festering wound was healing nicely on its own. It left no scar.

N.B. *Cabbage* is an extremely powerful healing agent and can become too stimulating, causing a feeling of irritation. If this occurs, sooth the area by switching to a *lettuce* poultice. I prefer *iceberg lettuce* for its large, easy to work with leaves. The leaves are prepared the same way, but only take a moment or two in the hot water to become translucent and pliable. You can alternate *lettuce* and *cabbage* poultices.

Jean Valnet removes the heavy midribs and

ALTERNATE METHODS FOR A CABBAGE POULTICE

then crushes the leaves one by one with a rolling pin or bottle. The white juice which oozes out is a powerful part of the healing. Be sure to capture as much as you can.
Valnet also recommends soaking the *cabbage*

leaves in warm *olive oil* for one half to one hour in the case of swollen, inflamed and sensitive conditions.

Maurice Messegue recommends an *olive*

oil maceration. He also uses a common household iron at the warm setting to iron the leaves until they are "like velvet".

Please read the section on Compound Poultices to read another story about the Power of *Cabbage*.

SIMPLE POULTICES

A simple poultice is made with a single herb. My stories about the power of *cabbage* certainly illustrate this point. In the chapter on herbal baths and soaks I give examples of the efficacy of using a single herb with marvelous results. Here are two examples of a simple poultice using fresh *comfrey*.

When I was living in the Smoky Mountains of North Carolina, I was thrown from a very tall horse onto a very hard gravel bank, severely jamming and spraining my left shoulder. I actually thought to myself "Here is a golden opportunity to test *comfrey*." (Only an herbalist would welcome an injury as an opportunity to learn something.)

I pounded fresh *comfrey* leaves into a pulp, using a large wooden bowl and large wooden pestle, and applied the pulp to my shoulder. I wrapped it first with some large *comfrey* leaves and then the usual clean, soft rags. It was awkward, but I managed. I changed this as often as I could, working one-handed. The relief after each fresh application was palpable. I experienced almost no pain, and in a week my shoulder was well, though still a little sore.

My second experience with a *comfrey* poultice came when I was living on San Juan Ridge with Rick Peltier. We lived in a 14' x 14' eccentric "owner built" (not by us) cabin with no plumbing and no electricity. Next to it was a half-finished barn which Rick enclosed and made into a workshop for *Medicine Flower*,

with my office up in the loft. In order to reach my office, I had to climb a heavy wood ladder leaning up against the edge of the loft.

Although I am fearful of heights, I learned to walk up and down the wooden ladder to the loft as if it were a staircase. Unfortunately, there was no cleat at the bottom of the ladder to hold it in place. One day, just as I had begun to walk down, the ladder slipped and I fell with my legs tangled in the rungs. I landed with my legs wedged awkwardly in the ladder on top of two large, heavy, sharp-cornered accordion cases.

After first aid, consisting of *Bach's Rescue Remedy* and *Reiki* to my adrenal glands (the treatment for shock), I instructed Rick in the making of a fresh *comfrey* poultice. He pounded the fresh, juicy leaves into a pulp, using my wooden bowl and pestle, then moistened the pulp with a little *apple cider vinegar* to facilitate absorption. This he bound onto my legs which were terribly and painfully bruised.

When the poultice became hot, indicating that it had drawn the heat of inflammation and shock out of my tissues, he applied a fresh poultice. This we kept up all day. The very next morning, when we unwrapped my legs, there was *no sign of bruising* except for around the edges where the poultice had not reached. Those areas were darkly black and blue and painfully tender. The area that had been under the poultice was in the pale yellow stage of a bruise almost healed.

This was a powerful testimonial to the efficacy of the fresh *comfrey* poultice, and the necessary practice of changing the poultice as soon as it becomes hot from drawing heat out of the injury.

The chapter on "The Power of *Cabbage*" gives two other examples of the use of a simple poultice. I also talk about *cabbage* in my discussion of Compound Poultices.

COMPOUND POULTICES

Many Moons have passed since I wrote the original article on "The Gentle Art of Poulticing" for *Mothering Magazine*, published in 1982. But there is so much more to say about poultices and other forms of using direct contact with herbs, rather than just the ingestion of herbal teas and tinctures. Here is more.

The account starting in the paragraph below was written in 2010.

Recently I had a chance to test the healing power of the poultice on a truly serious wound. The healing involved a series of compound poultices using a variety of herbs and materials, and was slow to come to completion. Some of this is because I am now 68 instead of 40, and my knees are arthritic, a condition of chronic pain and inflammation which impacts my immune system and my ability to heal as swiftly as I did when I was young. Because of all these variables, I thought it might be interesting to share the story of a healing journey which challenged me to use the more complex levels of my skills with the gentle art of poulticing.

About two weeks ago I tripped in a shopping mall parking lot and went down hard on my hands and knees on the rough, inhospitable road surface. My forward momentum dragged my left knee across the asphalt, creating a terrible wound. Before even trying to stand, I went into my purse for the medicines I always carry and took a dose of homeopathic *arnica*--as immediate first aid for the trauma and bruising. I also took a dropper of *Bach's Rescue Remedy*.

Kindly Samaritans helped patch me up so I could drive home. Once home I was horrified to see a knee that looked worse than any I'd produced at the age of 9, falling off my roller skates at full speed. I had a large area of deep wounding with ugly lacerations around the edges, tapering off to scrapes all around. Because of the unfortunate delay of more than an hour for first aid and driving time before I could begin treating it, the wound was already deep red with inflammation and the whole knee was painfully swollen, especially around the wound.

I began internal treatment with *garlic* (aka Russian penicillin). Every two hours the first day, then every four or so for the next two days, I chopped up a couple cloves of raw *garlic* and swallowed the little pieces with water. *Garlic* will purify the bloodstream in 4 minutes, and I wanted to keep my bloodstream full of *garlic's* antibiotic properties to get rid of any infection before it could take hold.

For **The First Stage poultice** I used a little *castor oil* mixed with powdered *wormwood, rosemary* and *goldenseal* (all strongly antiseptic). To this I added a clove of *garlic,* crushed in a press. This paste-like mixture I spread directly onto the open wound. The *garlic* burned like fire, but I did not want to take any chances with gangrene or blood poisoning. Over this I placed a *cabbage* poultice fashioned into a little pad. I prepared the *cabbage* by gently braising the leaves (divested of the hard central rib) until the leaves lost their opacity and were soft and limber. I laid the soft leaves on the wound, making a pad at least 4 layers thick. *Cabbage* is a powerful healer and I knew it would draw out toxins and stimulate a vigorous healing response.

I covered my herbal layers with a gauze pad, wrapped the knee with a nice clean, soft cotton flannel rag and taped it round and round.   Leggins kept the whole thing in place while moving and sleeping (the knee is a very mobile joint).   Later a nurse friend gave me a piece of stockinet that kept everything tidy.

After several days of this treatment plus *garlic* internally and high doses of anti-inflammatories like *turmeric, bromelain* (from pineapple) and *quercetin* (from oak bark), I could see granulation forming on the large, open surface and around the margins of the wound. This told me that new flesh was forming. The inflammation was almost gone.

At this point I felt the site was getting a little overstimulated, so I switched to **The Second Stage poultice** which consisted of a thick paste of *pascalite clay* covered with a pad of *iceberg lettuce* leaves, another compound poultice. *Lettuce* makes a calming, soothing, almost sedating poultice, which can be invaluable in certain stages of the healing process.

I prepared the *lettuce* in the same way as the *cabbage,* removing the midribs and gently heating the leaves in water. It only takes a few moments to soften the tender *iceberg lettuce* leaves. I still took *garlic* internally on occasion, and continued the internal anti-inflammatories, but at this point I stepped up regular icing of the knee by placing the ice bag on top of a cotton cloth covering the poultices. This really brought down the swelling. The dark red color of infection disappeared, and the edges of the wound began to pull together.   Granulation now had created healthy new flesh.

For variety, and for its demulcent, drawing, gently healing and nutritive qualities, I began **The Third Stage poultice** with a thick paste of hot water and *slippery elm bark* powder covered with a *lettuce* leaf pad. I continued to ice. Once or twice I mixed the powdered antiseptic herbs (*rosemary, wormwood* and *goldenseal*) in with the *slippery elm bark*. I kept up the internal anti-inflammatories and occasional internal disinfection.

At the end of about a week of this treatment, the wound had shrunk to less than half its original size and the ragged edges had pulled themselves together and filled in with new flesh. The edges reattached themselves to the sunken body of the wound, and everything looked nice and pink with white dots of new granulation popping up. Twenty years later there is a barely noticeable quarter inch diameter scar on my left knee.

Because the initial wound was so terrible, I went to my doctor who had only an over the counter antibacterial cream to offer. The cream did absolutely nothing, and the wound was so much worse the next morning it catapulted me into using my knowledge of poultices. I had never used any of these compound poultices before. I went purely by instinct and my knowledge of herbs. When I went to the doctor two weeks later, he couldn't believe his eyes, and even took a photograph of my knee!

One of reasons for writing this blow by blow description of how I used poultices in a specific situation was to document what I did. But another was to demonstrate that herbal healing takes place over time—there is no instant cure. Herbal medicine takes time and caring, a deep trust in the herbs, and a willingness to follow through a lengthy, repetitive protocol to bring the body into healing balance. A bit of curiosity is a good thing too.

HERBAL COMPRESSES, BATHS & SOAKS

There are other methods of getting the healing properties of herbs into the body via absorption through the skin. One of the simplest is the *cold compress*—a soft pad of cloth which has been saturated with an herbal brew or water to which a few drops of an essential oil have been added. Another is the herbal bath, requiring total immersion of the hands, feet or entire body in the herbal brew

The brew may be an *infusion* or a *decoction*. An *infusion* is made by pouring water just off the boil over the herbs, then covering and letting them steep for a period of time. A couple hours or overnight is best, but if time is of the essence, infuse for as long as possible. For a *cold infusion* simply steep the herb, covered, in cold water as long as possible. A *cold infusion* is used to preserve the most delicate or volatile properties of an herb, or when you want to dilute the raw juice of a plant. A *decoction* is used when preparing harder plant parts, like roots and bark (rarely seeds) by starting with the herbs in cold water, heating in a covered saucepan and then holding at a low simmer for a period of time. Excellent instructions for making these water based extractions can be found in Chapter Two of Juliette de Bairacli-Levy's *Herbal Handbook for Everyone.*

The Herbal Compress—A *cold compress* of *lavender* water with a couple drops of the essential oil is a remedy for headache, especially one brought about by stress or nervous strain. A *vinegar* compress was once the classic headache remedy, as well as being used for fresh bruises, strains and sprains. Brown paper, rather than cloth, was often used for a vinegar compress. I have no idea why brown paper was the preferred material in this case.

The Herbal Bath—The skin is the largest organ of elimination and absorption. It is sometimes referred to as "the third lung" because of its capacity to take in and release.

Maurice Messegue, the French traditional herbalist and simpler I mentioned earlier, used ONLY *herbal baths, compresses* and *hand and foot soaks.* He was famous for his herbal healings and was frequently called upon by French royalty and nobility for his services. He relates one experience where he saved the life of a member of the French nobility who was suffering from a life-threatening case of urinary retention by the simple application of a *cold compress* of the appropriate herb to the kidney area of the back.

There may be occasions where an *herbal bath* (which includes hand and foot soaks) may be the easiest, fastest and most appropriate way of getting the healing properties of herbs into the body. One of these occasions is when treating infants.

In a slender booklet I read on herbs used by the Paiute of Nevada I learned that every newborn baby was bathed in *mugwort* tea. I was initially puzzled until I remembered that *mugwort* has a favorable action on the liver, and that neonatal jaundice is a result of the newborn's liver not being able to break down bilirubin quickly enough.

Bilirubin is a yellow substance produced when red blood cells, which carry oxygen throughout the body, are broken down. The bilirubin is carried by the bloodstream to the liver and it is the liver's job to break it down so it can be eliminated through the baby's poop (ever notice that newborn poop is more yellow than brown?). Newborns have a very high level of red blood cells which are constantly being broken down and replaced, plus, the newborn's liver is not yet fully developed—it needs help.

Holy cow! I said to myself, the Paiute people are preventing neonatal jaundice in their newborn babies by this simple practice of bathing them in *mugwort* tea!

In fact, the action of *mugwort* in assisting the liver to do its job is so effective and well known, that in every Native American tribe I am aware of, women drink *mugwort* tea for the first three days of menstruation from their first Moon to their last. At the time of menstruation, a changing of the hormonal guards causes the release of blood from the uterus when the egg of the month is not fertilized. The liver needs help when the "getting ready for pregnancy" hormones are released to make way for a new configuration of hormones. Tribal women on their Moon are also forbidden to eat rich foods like meat and fat, which also give the liver more work to do. A lot of the distress around menstruation for women of the civilized world, from pimples to pre-menstrual syndrome and cramps, could be eliminated or ameliorated by the simple practice of drinking *mugwort* tea and abstaining from rich foods once a month from the first Moon to the last.

This would be especially important in the first years a young woman has begun her menses. The body is not yet used to the powerful, monthly purging of hormones when the body realizes there will be no baby this month. Ever notice how many teenagers get pimples if they eat chocolate right before and during their Moon? Ditto for other rich, fatty foods like cheese, French fries and all kinds of other such things.

THREE PERSONAL EXPERIENCES WITH HERBAL BATHS & SOAKS

My <u>first</u> experience with a successful full body herbal bath occurred in the 1980s when I was in practice as an herbalist on San Juan Ridge. A young couple called me late at night in great distress because their newborn infant had not pooped for the first three days of its life and they were justifiably worried.

It came into my mind that *fennel* was one herb that was potent yet gentle enough that it could be safely given to an infant. It is a *carminative*, meaning it helps expel gas from the lower digestive tract. I have used it when suffering terrible gas cramps and have always gotten immediate relief. My thought was that it would safely move the energy block in the baby's digestive system.

I advised the couple to make an infusion of *fennel* seeds (following Juliette's protocol for the Standard Brew) and bathe the baby in the *fennel* water. The next morning they called, ecstatic that their baby had "gotten going" in their words, and was following the normal newborn pattern of eat-sleep-poop.

My <u>second</u> experience with a successful herbal foot soak came in the 1990s when I was living and practicing as a healer in Nevada City. A young woman called me and said she had not slept for ten days and was beginning to hallucinate from lack of sleep. She was extremely environmentally sensitive and lived far out of town off the grid. She could only wear un-dyed clothing made from organic cotton and eat a very limited diet of clean, organic foods.

I asked her the questions I always asked of the people who called me (usually late at night): "What do you have in the refrigerator?" and "What do you have in your herb/spice rack?" Amazingly, she had three new heads of *iceberg lettuce* in the fridge, a food which popular belief says is devoid of nutritional and medicinal value. But I had faith that *all lettuce*, from the wild *Prickley Lettuce*, (*Lactuca serriola)* to the various varieties of cultivated *lettuce*, have sedative and analgesic (pain relieving) properties to varying degrees. Note: when wildcrafting, please do not confuse the "Compass Plant" (*Silphium lactinatum*) with *wild lettuce, (Lactuca*

serriola). The two plants are very similar and they are both members of the same family, *Asteraceae.*

I advised her to cut out the tough, hard core of each head, chop all of them coarsely and use them to make a decoction in a pot big enough so that she could make a foot soak that would cover her feet and her ankles. I also advised her to make an infusion of all three heads of *lettuce*, being careful not to heat the infusion above a very gentle simmer. I then suggested she soak her feet for at least 45 minutes to an hour before her intended bedtime and that she then drink the entirety of the brew in which all three heads of *iceberg lettuce* had been infusing. She called me the next morning and joyfully reported that she had experienced ten hours of the most delicious, restorative sleep. She continued to have normal sleep—the cycle of sleeplessness having been broken by the gentle, yet powerful action of one of the most despised plants in our edible plant pantheon. This taught me an important lesson—that when there is need, even the most common and overlooked herbs may be healing—and that *iceberg lettuce* is worthy of our respect.

My <u>third</u> experience was a personal one. In the early 2000s, the osteoarthritis in the lower joint of my right thumb where it joins the wrist became extremely painful and weak. The only solution medical doctors could offer was orthopedic surgery. Not only did surgery on my dominant hand not appeal to me, the surgeon assured me I would never play the guitar again!

So I called my wildcrafting and herbalist friend Ryan Drum, who lives on Waldron Island in the San Juan Islands off the coast of the state of Washington, for his always expert advice. Ryan is one of the best herbalists I know and a superlative wildcrafter. He gave me the recipes for hand soaks alternating *willow bark* and *fucus* (*bladderwrack*) seaweed. He suggested filling a neoprene glove or a pair of rubber boots with the herbal brew so I could walk around while the herbs were being absorbed through the skin of my hand or feet. But I found it easier to sit comfortably with a pot of hand soak on a stool next to my rocking chair. Here are the protocols exactly as Ryan dictated them to me.

HAND & FOOT SOAK PROTOCOLS

Willow Bark hand/foot soak

In a large pot put
   3 oz of willow bark
   3-1/2 quarts water
   Gently simmer 20 minutes, cover and let cool; reheat when you want to soak. A gentle simmer is approximately 180°F. I used a jelly thermometer to hold the simmer at the proper temperature.

Fucus (Bladderwrack or Bullwhip) Seaweed hand/foot soak

In a large pot put
   3 handfuls of fucus
   3-1/2 quarts water
Carefully heat to 140°F., cover and let cool; reheat when you want to soak.

Reheat all soaks to 140°F. every 48 hours to prevent spoilage. This is especially important with seaweed which is highly nutritious. Agar-agar, which is used in laboratory petri dishes to grow micro-organisms, is made of red algae.

VITAL: do not let fucus go down the drain.

Ryan said the **tiniest scrap** of seaweed let loose into your sewer or septic system, will grow into a giant nereocyctis kelp plant, attaining over 100 feet in length, causing permanent damage.

For a foot soak you will need a pot big enough to put your feet in, and enough herbal brew to cover your ankles. Try:
   4 oz bark per 1 gallon water/ or
   4 handfuls of fucus per 1 gallon water

Rule of thumb: 1 oz bark or 1 handful

of fucus per 1 quart water. Use similar proportions for other herbs. Adjust proportions if your herbs are extra fluffy and absorptive and you need more water. Barks and roots will need to be simmered whereas seaweed and tender herbs do not.

The Outcome

Although Ryan suggested alternating the two herbs every other day, I did not have enough plant material for this luxury. Therefore, I used the same batch of *willow bark* for a month before making another batch of *willow bark* soak. Heating the brew to 140°F every two days kept it from developing mold.

I was surprised when I developed a case of contact dermatitis. Even though I have never had a reaction to aspirin, this was an allergic reaction to the salicylates present in *willow bark*, doubtless due to the prolonged, daily exposure. I immediately switched to the *fucus* hand soak which speedily cleared up the dermatitis. The *fucus* felt divine, and I found myself squeezing it rapturously while soaking my right hand. The outcome was that the pain and weakness in the thumb of my right hand disappeared and has not returned to this day, well over ten years later!

N.B. As of this writing, it is twenty years later and the pain and weakness has not returned.

HOW TO MAKE THE BEST HERBAL SALVES

Herbal salves might be thought of as a kind of instant-poultice-in-a-jar, but there are important differences. A poultice is made in the moment, expressly to deal with a certain situation, and usually uses fresh plant material. A salve is an infusion of healing herbs in oil using very low heat. When the healing properties of the herbs have been extracted the oil is strained and just enough *beeswax* is added to give it body and preserve it. A poultice is thrown away once its purpose has been fulfilled whereas a salve is a way of preserving the healing properties of specific herbs for a very long time. As good as your salve may be, it will never achieve the same results as a good poultice. But the main advantage of a salve is that you make it once and it is always at hand and ready to use.

Choose the herbs for your salve according to the purpose you want it to serve. Do you want an emollient salve? Do you want an antiseptic salve? Do you want to promote healing? Reduce swelling and bruising? Ease cramps and muscle spasms?

This brings us into the complicated realm of formulation—the choosing of herbs to suit your purpose. The ability to create effective formulas is a profound skill, even an art. It is based partly on a deep knowledge of the multiple properties of each herb in your repertoire, partly on intuition, and partly on divine guidance. It is not the time or place to discuss the art of formulation, but I will say

the following: the ability to create good herbal formulas means knowing, *deeply* knowing, the multiple properties of any given herb—because *no herb does just one thing*.

Important: *you cannot study the herbs in your repertoire enough.* Study them in books, and study them by spending time with them and "getting" what they are about. If you are blessed, the plant will communicate with you and give you information beyond anything you can find in books. I cannot tell you how many times I have looked up *rosemary*. And if considering it for use I will look it up again—not in one, but in in several of my herb books, since each herbalist (and I only consider the herbalists who have had hands-on, clinical experience) may have different insights into a plant's properties.

Herbal salves are one of my specialties, and I am going to tell you *exactly* how to make the best salves.

Although I began my practice as an herbalist in 1969, it was not until I moved to the Smoky Mountains of North Carolina in 1972 that I believe I *truly* became an herbalist and a specialist in making herbal salves. I lived twelve miles up Caney Fork where the pavement ended, just about at the head of the hollow. I was deep in the mountains and the closest hospital was several hours away. I learned to care for myself and all the humans and animals for whom I felt responsible by using the healing herbs—the ones I grew in my garden and the ones I wildcrafted from the steep slopes surrounding my mountain home.

One day I was infusing a bunch of herbs in *olive oil*. My goal was to make an oil that would repel stinging insects like mosquitoes, gnats and deer flies. If you have ever been bitten by a deer fly you would want to do everything in your power to keep from being bitten again. I had already discovered that fresh Wormwood leaves, rubbed on my bare face, arms and shoulders, would keep the biting, stinging insects away from me for a period of time before I needed to reapply the fresh herb. Accordingly, my infusion contained Wormwood, Pennyroyal and a few other insect repelling herbs.

A couple days later when I went to the outhouse, I did not notice that a bunch of paper wasps had built a nest on the inside ceiling of the outhouse. The ceiling was quite low, so the top of my head brushed their nest. The next thing I knew I had five or six wasps in my hair biting my scalp repeatedly, while I watched with fascinated horror as a lone wasp crawled around on my wrist, biting out visible chunks of flesh. The next thing I knew I was back in the kitchen with my overalls flapping around my ankles, crying "Ow, ow, ow, ow ow". Instinctively I dipped my fingers in the herbed oil that was infusing near the warmth of the wood cook stove and rubbed it into my scalp. Fifteen minutes later the pain turned off like a lightbulb! *Gone!* Repeated applications that day prevented pain, itching and swelling. I knew I was on to something. A few more ingredients came to me from Spirit, and this is how *Elder Sisters Healing Herbal Salve* was born.

This is an example of a formulation that was "given" to me. I cannot explain to you how or why this combination of ingredients has such

miraculous effects. *Elder Sisters* is analgesic, anti-inflammatory, antiseptic and it promotes cellular regeneration. I have had hundreds of testimonials reporting miraculous results for a wide range of ills—from styes in the eye to severe burns to deep flesh wounds. It also has a mysterious ability to relieve certain kinds of pain.

The second formula I developed was a more deliberate formulation. I wanted a salve that would help stiff, sore muscles and painful joints, something that was also anti-spasmodic and therefore useful for everything from menstrual cramps to the severe spasms of a "charley horse". This salve infuses the chosen herbs in oil, and adds essential oils of specific herbs before the *beeswax* is added.

This is my *Penetrating Healing Herbal Salve* and I have hundreds of testimonials for everything from sinus congestion to severe arthritis. One woman claimed it dissolved a bone spur on her thumb!

If you are interested in **MEDICINE FLOWER HEALING HERBAL SALVES**, they are now made in Port Orford, Oregon by friends of mine. You can write to Linda Gordon c/o Medicine Flower, P. O. Box A, Port Orford, OR 97465, or email her at **medicine.flower72@gmail.com**.

HERBAL SALVE PROTOCOLS

Although I am not going to reveal my formulas, I am going to explain in detail the *exact* protocols I use. Three elements go into making great herbal salves: One—your formulation, Two—the quality of your ingredients, Three—following this protocol *exactly*. If kept in a cool place, your salves will last a very long time. If kept in the refrigerator, they will keep indefinitely. I have had people call me to say they have a jar of Elder Sisters or Penetrating Salve in the fridge and that the salves are still healing after 10-12 years.

Putting up the Salve
It is important that your herbs, oils and *beeswax* be of the best quality (organic for preference), and that all your utensils and receptacles are perfectly clean and dry. Remember that you are making medicine. If you are able to wildcraft, dry and store the herbs yourself, all the better. All herbs used in making a salve must be perfectly dried. If there is the tiniest bit of moisture in your herbs, you run the risk of mold. I learned this the hard way. As we famously know, oil and water do not mix. Even with the addition of *beeswax*, the herbed water will find its way to the top and become moldy.

Rule of thumb: For one ounce of herbs, use one cup of best oil, i.e. for each ounce of herbs by *weight*, use 8 ounces of oil by *volume*. Depending on the formula, I use organic, unrefined *olive oil* or organic, unrefined *sesame seed oil*. Unrefined *sesame seed oil* contains sesmoline, a natural preservative. I do not worry about adding preservative ingredients, even Vitamin E. In addition, many of the herbs in my formula are antiseptic and thus prevent spoilage.

Put the herbs in a large salve pot, add oil, stir and cover closely. An enameled pot without any nicks is perfect. Glass and stainless steel are also acceptable. *Do not use cast iron!* Place in an environment that will keep the salve "cooking" at 100 degrees 24/7 for *at least* one month. It is OK to go for two months.

Rick Peltier made a "salve cooker" for me that will hold two 2 gallon pots. It is a simple plywood box with a shelf salvaged from a small oven, which gives it two levels. A single *incandescent* light bulb keeps the temperature at 100 degrees and there is a rheostat to dim the bulb if it gets too warm. I keep an oven thermometer in the salve cooker to check the temperature. The new-fangled LED lightbulbs do not produce heat, so you will have to search for *incandescent* lightbulbs. People who need to keep baby chicks warm in an incubator also use *incandescent* lightbulbs, so you can find them if you try. When we lived on San Juan Ridge without electricity, Rick made me a giant salve cooker (capable of holding four two gallon batches of salve) from a 55 gallon drum heated with the burner unit salvaged from an old propane stove. When I first moved to town, the pilot light in my gas stove kept the oven at a steady 100 degrees Fahrenheit. The steady 100 degree heat, 24/7 for one to two months and *never* taking the lid off until the time is up are the most important factors.

Important: *Under no condition whatsoever open the lid of the salve pot until you are ready to strain, add beeswax and pour.* If you do, you will lose the delicate volatiles which contain important, subtle healing properties. The lengthy infusing time and inviolate rule of keeping the lid closed will insure that as many as possible of the healing virtues of the herbs go into the oil. Do not be tempted to lift the lid!

Straining the Herbs

You will need a second salve pot identical to the one you put the salve up in. Bind a more than adequate piece of flexible, fine meshed, non-metal screen to the second pot. Use strong twine and wrap it multiple times around the pot, *going both under and over the side handles.* You will be surprised at how heavy the oil soaked herbs are. I learned this lesson the hard way by having the whole mess plop down into the second pot. On top of the screen put a couple layers of the best quality, fine meshed cheesecloth. You might have to look in a fabric store as supermarket cheesecloth tends to be flimsy and not finely meshed enough.

Pressing gently, make a substantial indentation in the screen covering the mouth of the pot so that the mass of heavy, oily herbs has a safe place to rest and drain rather than bouncing off the taut surface of the screen and cheesecloth. Another lesson learned the hard way.

Now you can carefully and slowly pour the herbed oil through the mesh bound onto your pot, holding the mass of oily herbs back with a wooden spoon as long as possible. Then verrrrry gently and carefully spoon the mass of oily herbs into a mound on top of your mesh.

Let this drain for *at least* 24 hours, longer is better. Depending on the amount of salve material you are working with, you may be able to squeeze a little more herbed oil out of your oily mass with your hands. Just remember, if you squeeze too hard, you are going to get

more flecks of herbal matter in your herbed oil, and this residue will spoil the beauty and purity of your finished salves.

Now measure your yield of herbed oil and weigh the amount of *beeswax* you will need. **Rule of thumb: for each 8 ounces of herbed oil *by volume*, use 1 ounce of *beeswax by weight*.** This is just enough *beeswax* to make your salve "set up". It absolutely <u>will</u> <u>not</u> clog the pores of your skin, as some people fear.

Regarding *Beeswax*

If you are lucky enough to get your *beeswax* from a beekeeper, get *beeswax* that is dark with *propolis* instead of the "pretty" wax, because *propolis* is healing and antiseptic. The darker the *beeswax* the better. It will make your salve more powerful. When I was making salves regularly for the community I bought *beeswax* in 100# blocks from a beekeeper. The wax was a deep, dark olive green color with a divine fragrance. I had to purify the wax myself in order to strain out bees' legs and wings and other such things. Nowadays the places you find *beeswax* are craft stores for people who are making cosmetic creams and want *beeswax* that is almost white. Look for a local beekeeper. Just in case you need to purify your own wax, here is the way to do it.

Purifying *Beeswax*

If your *beeswax* comes from a beekeeper and is full of bee parts and other detritus, here is how to clean it for your salve. Chop some of the *beeswax* into very small pieces and add water enough to cover with a good inch or two to spare. The smaller the pieces of wax, the quicker they will melt into the water. Heat. Once everything has melted together, pour the *beeswax* and water into an old pie pan and let sit overnight. The next morning a cake of *beeswax* will have hardened and is now sitting on top of the water. Pour out the water. Now comes the fun part. With a chisel, scrape off the cruddy underside of your *beeswax* round, ridding it of bee body parts and other hive dirt. Your *beeswax* will be clean, yet dark with the healing and antiseptic properties of *propolis*.

Pouring the Salve

The night before you intend to pour the salve, you must take all the jars and caps you plan to use for your salve and sterilize them by pouring boiling water over them, or running the glass through the dishwasher (no soap needed). I use 2 ounce flint cream jars—they come in cases of 24 from Uline with caps included. *Don't put the caps in the dishwasher* as it will ruin the built in silicone seals. Make sure the jars are absolutely dry before using them for salves—remember that oil and water don't mix!

Put a layer of newspaper on the kitchen counter and set out your clean jars in neat rows. Be sure to leave good space between each jar so that the salve will cool and harden quickly. Set a single sheet of newspaper on top of the open salve jars to keep them clean while the salve is getting ready to pour.

Remember your rule of thumb. You are using **one ounce of *beeswax* by *weight* for one cup (8 ounces) by *volume* of herbed oil**. Chop and shave the *beeswax* into small pieces. The smaller the pieces of wax the sooner they will melt in the oil, which will affect the quality of the resulting salve. It is to your benefit and the quality of your salve to use low heat for the shortest period of time. After all the trouble you've gone to, it would be a pity to burn off the subtle healing qualities of your herbed oil by letting it get too hot for too long.

Using a small measuring cup, pour molten salve (herbed oil plus melted *beeswax*) into your jars. Be sure to leave enough head space in your jars for your top pour the next day. I

pour to just barely over the shoulder of the jar. Also be sure to reserve enough molten salve to use for the top pour. Replace the single sheets of newspaper on top of the jars and divert yourself until the salves have hardened all the way through. The further apart the jars of salve stand, the more quickly they will harden.

The Top Pour

Oddly, when the salve hardens in the jar, you will find either little craters in the center or circular cracks on the surface of the salve. Don't ask me why this happens. Now gently reheat the remaining salve in your big pot and from your measuring cup, gently pour the thinnest film of barely melted salve over the top of the salve in each jar—you don't want the molten salve to be so hot it melts the salve that's already in the jar. This time, when it hardens, it will present a perfectly smooth, beautiful surface. Cover with the sheet of newspaper and wait until salves are well cooled before putting the caps on. You will find you have to tighten the caps again before putting your salves away in the cardboard cases. Be sure to *label* the outside of the box with the date and name of the salve.

Keeping Records

This may seem boring but it's important. I keep a three ring binder with the records of every single batch of salve I've ever made. In the beginning of each different salve section in the binder I give the formula—the exact amount of each herb in the formula to add to two gallons of oil. I always make salve in two gallon batches. You will adjust the amount for your practice.

For each batch of salve I make I record the date, and reiterate the formula and the amount of oil. After that I record the date I put up the herbs in the oil, the date I took the salve pot out of the cooker, the yield of herbed oil produced after straining the herbs out and the calculation for the amount of *beeswax* needed. Finally, I record the total yield of the batch in numbers of jars.

It is absolutely critical to have a good scale if you are going to make good salves. I bought a triple beam balance scale when I started out, but it has the annoyance of having to translate ounces into grams in order to get the correct ratio of *beeswax* to herbed oil. A good kitchen scale which will give you accurate measurements in ounces is probably easier. I have been using the triple beam for so many years, I find that I get the best results when I weigh out the *beeswax* by grams on this particular scale.

Cleaning Up

This first time I made a big batch of salves was almost the last time I made a big batch of salves. Cleaning salve (herbal oil plus *beeswax*) off the inside of an enamel salve pot is difficult, discouraging and almost impossible unless you have this secret ingredient—**_Alconox_**. *Alconox* is a laboratory glass cleaner. *First*, it has almost no foam or bubbles. Cleaning products are designed to make bubbles because it gives the user a feeling that the product is powerful—but bubbles are not what cleans. *Second*, it leaves virtually no residue on the glass or whatever you are cleaning. You can easily see how important this is for a laboratory cleaning product—the last thing you want is residue of soap or detergent on your test tubes and petri dishes. *Third*, it has fabulous cleaning ability—a little goes a long way. My scientific and ethnobotanical friend, Dale Pendell, turned me on to it. Without *Alconox*, I doubt I would have developed *Medicine Flower* and become a salve maker. Cleaning up would have defeated me. You will be amazed at what even a small amount of *Alconox* can do.

When you have finished making your salve, wipe down the inside of your salve pot to get as much salve off the oily, beeswaxy surfaces as possible. Depending on the formula, of course, you can wipe out the pot with your hands and anoint yourself all over. Lovely for the skin. Or use a paper towel. If you have a wood burning stove, this oily-waxy paper burns nicely. Then put some *Alconox* in your vessel, fill with super hot water and let soak for a while. Then clean the pot as usual.

I even clean the cheesecloth that I lay over the screen to strain the herbed oil. I soak the cheesecloth in a strong *Alconox* and very hot water solution, dunking and squeezing the cheesecloth many times and then rinsing and squeezing many times in hot water. Repeat. By the time I am done with the cheesecloth, it is not even slightly oily, and barely smells of the herbed oil. It will have only the slightest discoloration from the herbs. I have been using the same high quality cheesecloth for years.

The first time I bought *Alconox* I had to go to a laboratory supply place in Sacramento. Now, you can probably get it on-line like everything else. If you get it from Amazon or any other similar source, be sure that the product is not only called *Alconox*, but that it is made and sold by *Alconox*.

USING SALVES IN LIEU OF POULTICES

Elder Sisters Healing Herbal Salve

Here are a couple examples of how I have used *Elder Sisters* in the same way as I would a poultice. *Elder Sisters* is antiseptic, analgesic, anti-inflammatory and promotes cellular regeneration, among other mysterious and almost magical properties.

Once I poured boiling oil over my left hand, creating a second degree burn. I patted my hand dry with a paper towel and then slathered *Elder Sisters* all over the burned area. I did not first rinse my hand in icy cold water—a popular burn remedy that actually makes things worse. Any moment wasted increases oxidation, increasing the severity of the burn. And water contains oxygen (H_2O) also increasing oxidation. I sat down with a book. At first, my conscious mind was filled with the pain in my left hand. After a little while, maybe fifteen or twenty minutes, I found myself reading enjoyably and suddenly remembered that I had burned myself. The pain was gone. I applied *Elder Sisters* three or four more times before bed. After the last generous application I wrapped my hand gently in a soft, clean flannel rag.

When I woke up the next morning there was absolutely no sign of a burn. No redness, no blisters, no wrinkling of the skin. I continued applications of *Elder Sisters* for the next day or two. There was and is no sign that my hand was ever burned.

On another occasion, I got a call from a friend who had fallen off the roof of his RV entangled in his ladder, and had ripped a mighty strip of skin and flesh off his leg from knee to ankle.

I applied a generous amount of *Elder Sisters* salve directly onto the raw, wounded flesh. The idea behind a generous application is that it allows the salve to continue to be absorbed into the body without disturbance. I then tenderly wrapped his leg with cheese cloth, then with clean, soft rags and finally with an ace bandage to keep it all in place. I told him not to unwrap or disturb the bandaging in any way. After one week, we unwrapped the bandages and were greeted by the vision of pink, healthy flesh with little islands of granulation, indicating that tissue regeneration was already underway. He said there had not been a single moment of pain or itching. I gave him a couple jars of *Elder Sisters* to keep up the treatment. His leg healed without scarring.

Penetrating Deep Gentle Warming Herbal Salve

This salve I created specifically for stiff, sore muscles and joints. The addition of essential oils makes it especially powerful. It does not need to be applied lavishly—a thin film will do. And it must be kept away from the eyes or any mucous membrane.

I have not had an opportunity to use this salve in lieu of a fresh herb poultice, but I would not hesitate to use it as I would an *onion* poultice or *mustard* plaster in the case of seriously congested lungs, especially if I had nothing else.

When I moved from the Ridge to Nevada City in 1988, my chiropractor became interested in this salve and started using it in lieu of his ordinary ultrasound gel. He said it made it so much easier to adjust his patients because the salve relaxed muscle tension, dissolving any resistance to the adjustment. A massage therapist told me something similar—that using *Penetrating Salve* with his clients swiftly relaxed tense muscles and made it easier for him to "get in" to do his work.

Most of the testimonials for this salve are from people suffering from arthritis and other forms of musculo-skeletal pain and spasm. An eighty year old woman has her husband massage her all over with *Penetrating Salve* every morning—otherwise, she claims, she would not be able to get out of bed and move around. Another woman, in the course of massaging *Penetrating Salve* into her husband's sprained and separated shoulder three times a day for four weeks, claimed that the bone spur in her right thumb that was keeping her from holding a paint brush (she is an artist),

had dissolved and has never returned. I have had athletes tell me they anoint themselves with *Penetrating Salve* before a workout or competition, because it enables them to begin exertion with warm, relaxed muscles, thus preventing all kinds of injury, and post-workout soreness and fatigue.

In Conclusion
A salve *is not* like a poultice, compress or bath in that the herbs used are not fresh and prepared specifically for the problem of the moment. But a salve *is* like a poultice in that the healing herbal properties are applied directly to and absorbed through the skin. Each method—poultice, compress, fomentation, bath or salve—has its strengths. It will be well worth your while to learn how to work with each one of these healing modalities.

GRANNY'S SPIRIT GATE TEA

3 parts — Of *Hawthorn Berries*, gathered bright and sweet after first frost, dried well and ground in a hand mill

2 parts each — Of *Raspberry Leaf* and *Strawberry Leaf* gathered before the berries form and take the virtue from the leaves

1 part — Of *Borage Tops* with flowers in full color

1 part — Of tiny fragrant *Cecile Brunner Rosebuds*

1 part — Of *Stinging Nettle* leaf

1 part — Of *Rosemary Needles*

1 part — Of *Fennel Seeds*

1 part — Of *Licorice Root*, snipped into tiny bits

Crush the leaves very, very gently in your hands and mix together with the ground berries, the roots, needles and seeds. This tea will open the heart and cheer the spirits.

In making Medicine as in making your life— let all ingredients be of the very best quality. Handle lightly with love.

Use care and attention to detail.

Ask for it to be good.

Find your own way.

Dedicate the merit of your work for the benefit of All Sentient Beings.

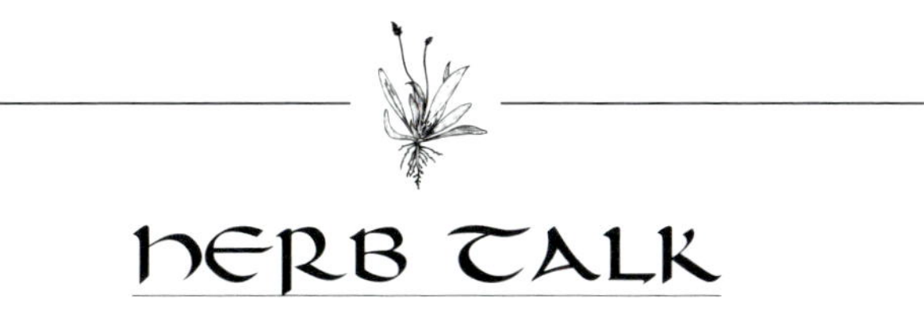

ΗΕRB ΤΑLΚ

INTRODUCTION TO "HERB TALK"

The following section consists of a series of little columns I wrote in 1981 for *The Independent*, Nevada City's weekly newspaper (now defunct). A friend of mine cut out each article and glued it to a piece of paper, creating a booklet, the original of which I have donated to the Searls Library—the archive for the Nevada County Historical Society. These newspaper articles are a very small part of the work I did for the three year grant from the California Arts Council to be a folklorist/folksinger in the community. These little articles grew out of a weekly radio program called *Herb Talk*, which I did for KVMR, our community volunteer radio station.

Because these are newspaper clippings, there is no way I can correct typos and mend other blemishes in the copy. Nor can I straighten out the way each article was glued onto the blank sheet of paper. Please accept these clippings as they are, and enjoy the tidbits of herbal information they contain.

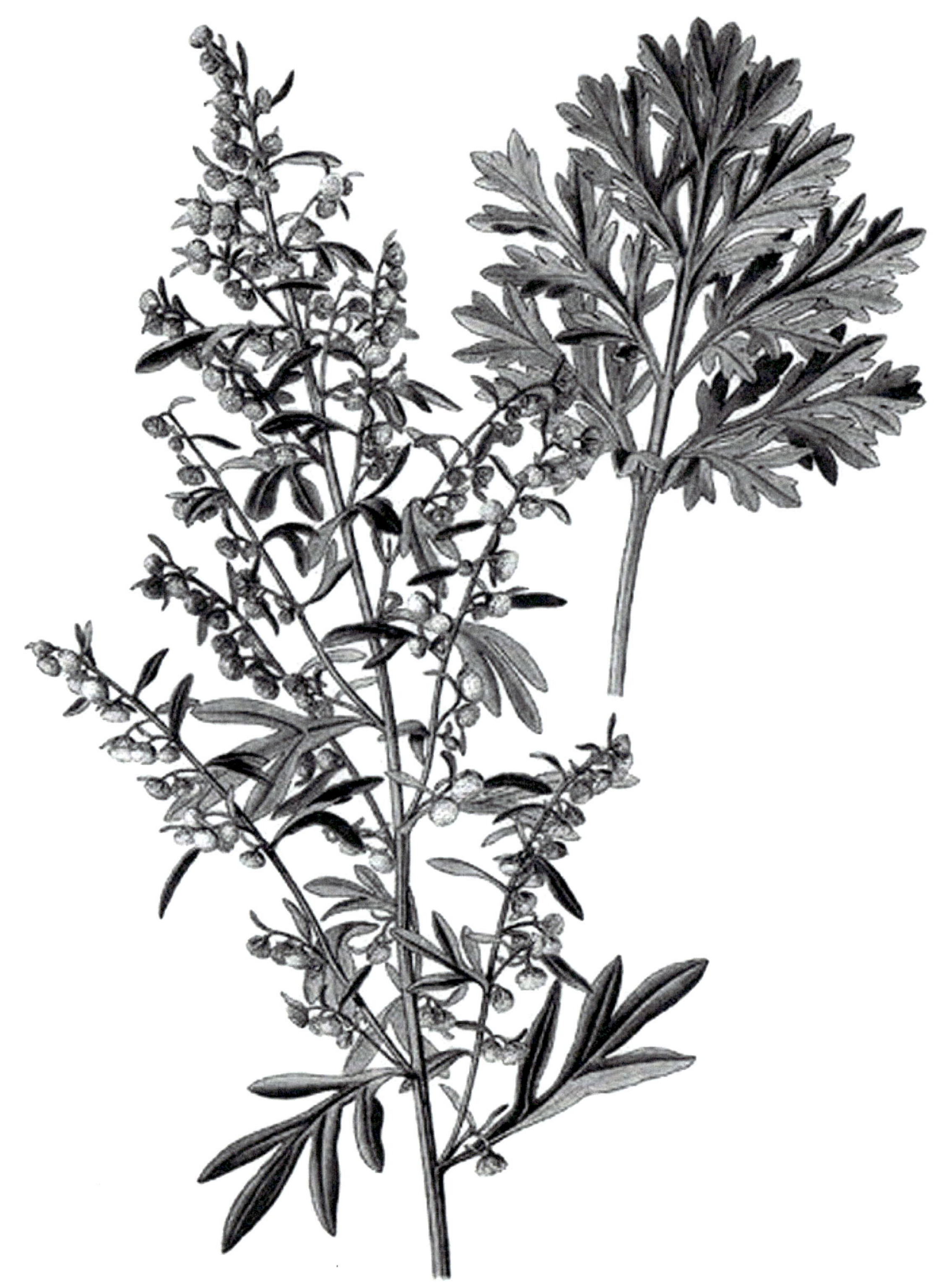

Artemisia Absinihium L.

Wormwood

HERB TALK

By Marina Bokelman

Published in the *Independent*

From June 10, 1981 to December 23, 1981

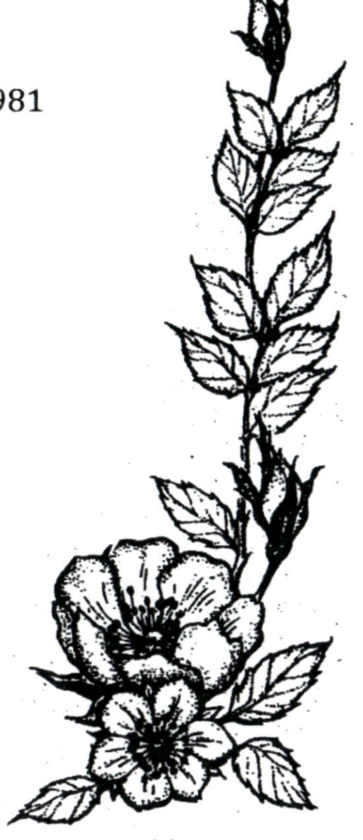

Wild Rose

INTRODUCTION

In 1980 I got involved with KVMR, Nevada City's community radio station. I had my own traditional folk music show, *Folk Plus* (later *Buckdancer's Choice*), and I was also a weekly guest on Jima Abbott's *Afternoon Show*. I did a forty-five minute segment called *Herb Talk*. My practice was to focus on common edible and medicinal herbs and weeds, and on the wild plants of our foothill area. I also touched on the ailments and issues of each season.

In 1981 I was asked to do a weekly *Herb Talk* article for each issue of *The Independent*, Nevada City's independent newspaper. Each article reflected, in condensed form, the topic of my radio *Herb Talk* for the week the newspaper was published.

This booklet contains the 17 articles published in the Independent from June 10, 1981 to December 23, 1981, plus *Health Talk/Herb Talk*.

In 1984 Dr. Jeff Kane interviewed me for one hour on his weekly KVMR program, *Health Talk*. *Health Talk/Herb Talk* is a highly condensed excerpt from that interview. It appeared in *Airnotes*, the Fall 1984 edition of KVMR's quarterly Program Guide and Newsletter.

CONTENTS
Scotch Broom Revisited
Manzanita
Yerba Santa
Mullein
Insect Repellants
Insect Bites and Stings
Fennel
Lettuce
The Rose Family
Mugwort
The Almond
Apples
Herbs as Food & Medicine
Horseradish
Cabbage
Herbal Antiseptics—Myrrh
Holly & Ivy

ADDENDUM
Health Talk/Herb Talk

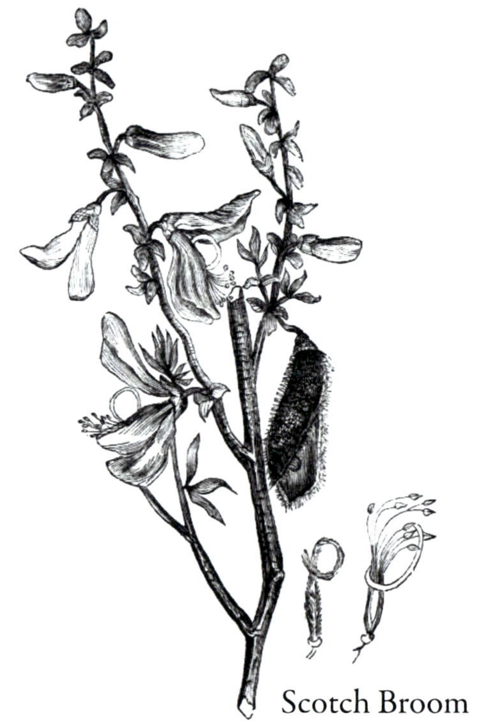

Scotch Broom

May all Beings Benefit

Herb Talk: Scotch broom revisited

by Marina Bokelman

Elaine McPherson's article on Scotch Broom in the April 29 Independent got me searching for more information about this beautiful but unpopular plant.

Broom *(Cytisus scoparius)* was considered a useful plant in times past. Pliny and Virgil wrote about it under the name of *Genista,* and it is mentioned in all the earliest published herbals, beginning in 1485.

Interestingly, this hardy member of the legume family can be classed as food, medicine or poison, depending on which part of the plant is used and how far the growing season is advanced.

The unopened buds are edible, pickled like capers in vinegar or salt. Broom buds were once considered such a delicacy that they appeared on three separate tables at the coronation feast of James II. The flowers were eaten as an appetizer.

Medicinall, the tender young tips of the flowering branches are used, gathered early in spring. Broom tops are diuretic and cathartic and were mostly used for chronic dropsy. It is still listed as an "official" drug in the *sparteine* increases in all parts of the

As the season advances, the alkaloid *sparteine* incrases in all parts of the plant, greatly increasing its toxicity. In large doses Broom causes vomiting and purging, heart damage and respiratory paralysis. Death may result. Its action is very similar to Hemlock, the plant poison used to execute Socrates.

Obviously, this is not a plant to be used except by a medical practitioner. If you are looking for a mild diuretic, try corn silk, carrot juice or raw asparagus. Much safer and tasty too.

Even more interesting are Broom's historic connections. Richard the Lion Heart depicted the Broom flower on his Great Seal, and Henry II also adopted it, the medieval name *Planta genista* giving the name Plantagenet to his family line. Among peasants, Broom was considered a charm against witchcraft and bouquets of the brilliant yellow blooms were carried by wedding guests to ward off evil from the young couple.

Broom has also had many economic uses. It was used to make brooms and baskets, to thatch cottages, dye wool, tan leather, and brew beer (the tender young tops were used to impart a bitter flavor before hops were discovered) among other things. Add to this the facts that it fixes nitrogen in the soil (being a legume) and prevents erosion by holding the soil together, and it is hard to keep thinking of Scotch Broom as an unmitigated pest. Like all of us, it has its faults and its good points.

Manzanita

Now is the time to gather Manzanita—when the strong young leaves are coming out and before the plant begins to put all its energy into ripening the nutritious red berries.

These berries are so appreciated by bears that the genus is called *Arctostaphylos,* which means "Bear Grape" in Greek. The familiar sturdy shrub, with red bark and dull grey-green leaves is *Arctostaphylos manzanita.* The common name means "Little Apple" in Spanish.

Like its close relative Uva Ursi (Kinnikinnick), Manzanita is a diuretic and has a mild disinfecting quality useful in inflammations of the urinary tract and in cases of bladder stone. The herb is effective as a tea (1 tsp. of the chopped leaves to 1 cup boiling water) or as a tincture (20-30 drops). The leaves of the Manzanita are quite astringent and a strong infusion (perhaps mixed with Yerba Santa) is said to give relief from poison oak.

Caution should be exercised in using this plant internally as large or frequent doses may irritate the intestinal tract. Also, Manzanita should be avoided by pregnant women as it constricts the flow of blood to the uterus.

The berries of the Manzanita were used by native Californians to make a sweet-tart cider, which could also be fermented into "hard cider" and vinegar. In fact, Manzanita was so prized as a source of food and drink that individual families could own the right to harvest from a specific patch of bushes. Some tribes even held a dance and Big Eat at the time of the Manzanita harverst.

Marina Bokelman may be heard on **Herb Talk** every Monday at 5 p.m. on KVMR.

Herb Talk: Yerba Santa

If you look out your car window while driving along the freeway from Nevada City to Grass Valley, you will notice a low shrubby evergreen plant with dark green, rather leathery looking lance-shaped leaves. If you are driving very slowly you will see that the leaves and stems of this rather straggly shrub are covered with a slightly sticky varnish-like resin. This plant, almost unnoticeable except when the tall stalks with terminal clusters of bluish purple funnel-shaped flowers shoot up, is one of the great healing plants of California.

This plant was so prized by native Californians that the Spanish missionaries, who learned the use of the plant from the Indians, called it *Yerba Santa,* meaning Blessed or Holy Herb.

Also called Tar Week or Mountain Balm, this aromatic, balsamic plant is a specific remedy for problems of the respiratory system, including asthma, bronchitis, laryngitis and chest colds. It is a mild expectorant and decongestive.

Native Californians also used it as a smoke and chewed the slightly bitter leaves to purify the breath and allay thirst.

Spanish padres quickly learned to use this herb and no mission in California was without its extract of Yerba Santa, tinctured in whiskey. The plant was listed as an official drug in the United States Pharmacopoeia from 1894 to 1947 and was picked up by the National Formulary in 1947.

Safe dosage of Yerba Santa is 1 tsp. of the crushed leaves to 1 cup of water, taken in half cup doses, 2 to 4 times daily. Of the tincture, 10 to 30 drops in a glass of water is sufficient.

Remember—never gather Yerba Santa, or any medicinal herb, by the side of the road, no matter how prolific it may be. Not unless you want to take a heavy dose of automobile emissions along with your herbs!

Marina Bokelman may be heard on HERB TALK, every Monday at 5 p.m. on KVMR, 89.5 FM.

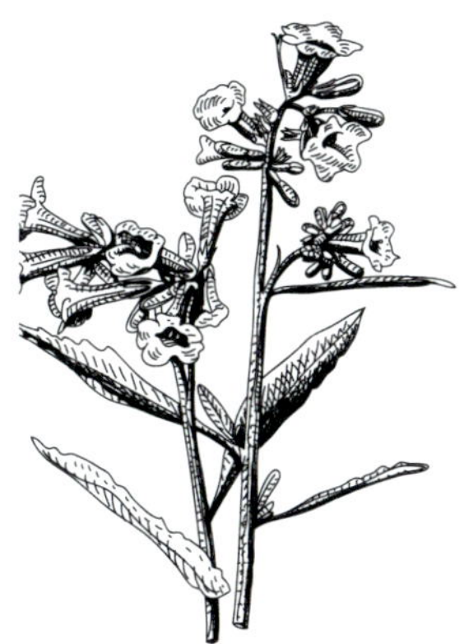

Yerba Santa

Herb Talk:
MULLEIN

By Marina Bokelman

One of the more impressive midsummer displays is made by Mullein *(Verbascum thapsus)* with its thick yellow-tipped flower stalk rising 4 to 6 feet above the large basal leaves. Once seen up close this plant is never forgotten. The pale green leaves and stem are densely covered with short, soft hairs, giving the entire plant a fuzzy texture and appearance, reflected in the common names Blanket Leaf, Felt Wort, and Flannel Plant.

Mullein favors waste places and soil distributed by clearing, ploughing and burning. It is easily tamed and thrives under cultivation. In England, in fact, it is widely grown as a garden ornamental.

Hippocrates and Dioscorides, our earliest herb writers, praised Mullein as a remedy for all ailments of the chest--congestion, coughs, bronchitis, asthma and consumption. According to the National Formulary (1916-1936), its properties are pectoral, anodyne, demulcent and antispasmodic.

When boiled in milk, the leaves are astringent, giving relief in diarrhoea and dysentery. The leaves soaked in hot vinegar make a poultice for swollen glands, and an oil made from Mullein blossoms (which are mildly sedative) is a popular remedy for earache. The dried leaves are combined with other pectoral herbs and smoked for asthma.

Any preparation of Mullein for internal use must be carefully strained through a fine sieve or cloth as the tiny hairs can irritate the throat--causing the cough rather than relieving it.

Other common names for Mullein are Candlewick and Our Lady's Taper, giving us a clue to its earlier uses. In ancient England Mullein down was dried and used in tinder boxes or rolled into wicks for oil lamps before cotton was introduced. In Elizabethan times the entire stalk was dried, then soaked in tallow and used as a torch.

The blossoms of this versatile plant were used to dye wool green or brown (depending on the mordant used) and the seeds were used by poachers to stun fish. And, like many other pharmacologically active plants with brilliant yellow blossoms--such as Scotch Broom and St. John's Wort--Mullein was once used all over Europe and Asia as protection against the workings of magic.

Marina Bokelman can be heard on Herb Talk every Monday at 5:00 p.m. on KVMR, 89.5 FM.

HERB TALK

By Marina Bokelman

Summertime is bug time. The deer fly with its swept-back bomber wings and painful nip menaces the home gardener. Nesting wasps circle the nervous carpenter. Mosquitoes pester everyone. And then there are the fleas.

There *are* alternatives to Cutters and Black Flag. Many of the aromatic herbs, rich in essential oils, are effective insect repellants. Wormwood *(Artemisia absinthium),* pennyroyal *(Mentha pulegium),* rue *(Ruta graveolens),* rosemary *(Rosmarinus officinalis),* southernwood *(Artemisia abrotanum),* and eucalyptus *(Eucalyptus spp.)* all have insect repelling qualities. And unlike citronella (commercially extracted from *Cymbopogam nardus)* these pleasantly pungent herbs will not repel other human beings!

If you are lucky enough to have any of these herbs growing in your garden, try crushing and rubbing the fresh leaves on your skin for temporary protection. Or, if you are more ambitious, make your own insect repellant oil.

Take a couple handfuls of your fresh pungent aromatics, in any combination, chop the leaves and place in a glass jar, barely covering the herbs with any cold-pressed vegetable oil. Cap tightly and let sit in the sun for 7 to 10 days, shaking daily. Squeeze out the spent herbs and discard, repeating the whole process with fresh herbs until a highly aromatic oil results. Bottle and use as you would any insect repellant.

An even simpler repellant can be made by adding one ounce of pure essential oil of pennyroyal to three ounces of cold-pressed vegetable oil. Bottle and use. This oil can also be diluted with water and used as a flea spray for pets. The Latin name for pennyroyal means "flea mint" (mentha-mint, pulegium-flea), reflecting its power to repel these particular insects.

Please remember that essential oils are highly concentrated and powerful and should be treated with caution. Essential oil of pennyroyal in particular should never be taken internally.

Marina Bokelman may be heard on HERB TALK, every Monday at 5 p.m. on KVMR, 89.5 FM.

HERB TALK

INSECT BITES & STINGS

By Marina Bokelman

Insect bites are a fact of life in the summertime and a painful reminder that we no longer live in the Garden of Eden.

The all-too-familiar symptoms of pain, itching, inflammation and swelling are an allergic reaction to whatever it is that particular insect injects into its host or prey. The severity of the reaction varies from person to person.

No matter what kind of bug bites you, the secret is to act quickly. Immediate treatment can prevent much of the expected discomfort and swelling.

There are many herbs useful as topical first-aid treatments for insect bites and stings. Plantain *(Plantago major)* and dock *(Rumex crispus)* are the two poultice herbs most commonly used to soothe bites. Simply pulp the fresh green leaves by pounding or chewing and place the resulting moist pad of herb over the bite. Garlic *(allium sativum)*, pounded in a mortar or mashed with a garlic press, is useful first-aid remedy for bites, and has the advantage of being right there on the kitchen shelf.

Interestingly, many of the herbs used to repel insects are effective for treating bites and stings. The fresh green leaves of wormwood *(Artemisia absinthum)*, rosemary *(Rosmarinus officinalis)* and rue *(Ruta graveolens)* can be pulped and bound over the area. Or try making an "herbed oil" of these plants (follow directions for insect repellant oil in THE INDEPENDENT, July 29, 1981) to have on hand or to take camping. The essential oils in the pungently aromatic herbs seem to help neutralize the toxins in the sting while relieving pain and inflammation. Rue was even blessed by the prophet Mohammed after gypsies used this herb to cure him of a poisonous scorpion sting.

Another kitchen remedy worth remembering is meat tenderizer! It contains a protein-digesting enzyme which helps break down those allergy-provoking substances injected under the skin. As with all bug bite remedies, this must be used immediately for maximum effectiveness.

Some people have such severe allergies to certain insect bites that medical treatment is required. If you are such a person, don't risk substituting an herbal remedy for the treatment recommended by your health care provider. But, for the rest of us, prompt use of simple herbal remedies may make it unnecessary to itch and bear it when insects bite.

Marina Bokelman may be heard on HERB TALK, every Monday at 5 p.m., on KVMR 89.5 FM.

HERB TALK
Fennel

by Marina Bokelman

Fennel *(Foeniculum officinale)* is one of the least known of all the common, useful herbs. It is in bloom all over California at this time of year--the tall plants with dark green feathery leaves and small yellow flowers in umbels forming dense clumps on dry banks near parking lots, along roadsides, and at odd corners in yards and vacant lots. In appearance it is very like a giant dill plant. Chew the leaves, however, and you will at once recognize the taste of licorice, a flavor shared by anise *(Pimpinella anise)*, with which fennel is often confused. Actually, fennel, anise and dill are all members of the Umbelliferae Family and share similar medicinal properties.

Fennel was a favorite culinary and medicinal herb of the ancient Romans who carried it from its native Mediterranean to every corner of the Roman Empire. They even developed a tender garden variety *(Foeniculum dulce)* which sometimes appears in California supermarkets as Florence Fennel.

Fennel's chief use is for all manner of digestive complaints. The seeds can be chewed to relieve gas pains and are toasted and served after dinner in India for this purpose. Fennel seed tea is also a favorite remedy for infant colic and other digestive upsets of the newborn.

Along with catnip and dill, fennel may be given to infants and children with confidence.

Not only is it versatile and mild in all its actions, it is pleasant tasting too! Nursing mothers may also drink fennel seed tea with benefit as it will increase the flow of milk.

Fennel has been listed in the National Formulary and United States Pharmacopoeia as an official medicine plant. It is mildly sedative (good for teething infants), antispasmodic (useful in cough syrups and for lung problems), aperient (mildly laxative), preventive of griping (therefore added to strong laxative blends), and tonic to the liver and gall bladder. It also makes an excellent complexion lotion and eyewash. To soothe and clear sore eyes: place over the eyes cotton balls soaked with a cooled tea made of equal parts fennel seed, elder blossoms *(Sambucus spp.)* and eyebright *(Euphrasia officinalis)*. Renew when the cotton feels warm to the touch.

As if all this weren't enough, fennel is the essential ingredient in Swedish limpa bread, German pfefferneuse and Italian sausage (of course) and is used in making dozens of cordials and liqueurs.

Since fennel is so inexpensive, common, easy to cultivate, medicinally versatile, mild, safe and tasty, how come it's not famous?

Marina Bokelman can be heard on HERB TALK, every Monday at 5 p.m. on KVMR, 89.5 FM.

HERB TALK:
The Rose Family

Certain traits are said to "run in the family" and this is true of plant families as well. Related plants are biochemically similar and may therefore have similar properties when taken as food or medicine.

Take the *Rosaceae* for example. Members of this **Family include the Rose,** Strawberry, Raspberry, Blackberry, Cherry, Plum, Peach, Pear, Apple and Almond. **All these plants are highly nutritious; they sustain** life and promote health. And because they are also tender **and tasty, we have adopted** them as foods. Unfortunately, these familiar plants are so often thought of in terms of their beauty, fragrance and taste, it is forgotten that these Rose relatives have healing properties.

Let us look at the first four on the list: the Rose *(Rosa spp.)*, Strawberry *(Fragaria vesca)*, Raspberry *(Rubus idaeus, Rubus strigosus)*, and Blackberry *(Rubus fruticosus)*. All four of these plants are nutritious, refrigerant (cooling the body temperature), astringent, laxative, purifying to the blood and tonic to the nerves and female reproductive system. All parts of these plants are medicinal—from root to fruit.

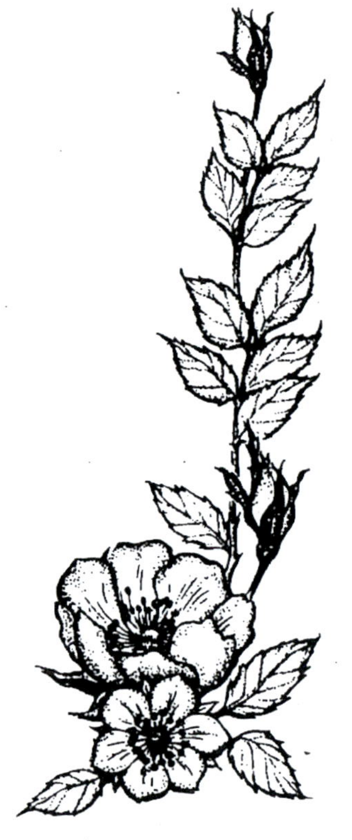

The differences between the four are in degree and emphasis.

The Rose is the gentlest astringent, a brew of the petals being an ancient beauty aid for the complexion. The same mild astringency makes Rose petal tea useful as a douche. The Rose is tonic to the heart, brain and lungs as well as being strengthening to the ovaries and uterus. The Dog Rose *(Rosa canina)* reminds us that the Rose (as a blood purifier) was an ancient remedy for dog bite. The fruits of the Rose—the hips — are well known for their high vitamin C content.

The Strawberry is the most powerfully refrigerant and purifying to the blood. In fact, the "strawberry rash" experienced by some people is a result of this herb's powerful cleansing action which drives acids from the system through the skin faster than the body's other eliminative systems can process them. The fruits are rich in minerals, especially iron, phosphorus, calcium and bromide, and are an excellent remedy for anemia and nervous conditions. Levulose is the form of sugar in Strawberries, making them an acceptable sweet for diabetics.

The Raspberry excels as a pregnancy herb, the high *fragrine* content being responsible for its tonic effect on the entire female reproductive system. Taken daily during pregnancy it strengthens the uterus and relieves morning sickness. During childbirth it facilitates an efficient labor, and immediately afterwards helps bring down the placenta. A tea of the astringent leaves is a remedy for infant diarrhea. The fruits of the Raspberry plant are also rich in minerals and levulose.

The Blackberry shares the basic family characteristics but is the most astringent of **the lot. A brew of the tan**nin-rich leaves and root bark **makes a useful gargle, mouth** wash, skin cleanser and douche. An old-fashioned remedy for "summer complaint" in children (diarrhea) is a honey syrup made with 1 part ripe Blackberries and 1 part unripe Blackberries.

So **do** eat the Roses. For pleasure, for nourishment, as preventive medicines and as delicious and delightful **remedies when called upon** for healing.

Marina Bokelman may be heard with HERB TALK every Monday at 5 p.m. on KVMR, 89.5 FM.

HERB TALK

Lettuce

Prickly Lettuce *(Lactuca scariola)* is one of the more interesting-looking roadside plants. It is erect, up to four feet tall, covered with prickles, and has deeply lobed leaves resembling, from a distance, black oak leaves. These leaves, which alternate along the stem, hold their flat surfaces perpendicular to the ground, unlike most other plants. As a further idiosyncracy, Prickly Lettuce orients its leaves along the north-south axis, giving rise to the popular name "Compass Plant."

The generic name "Lactuca" comes from the Latin word for "milk" and describes the thick, bitter white sap which Prickly Lettuce shares with all members of the lettuce tribe.

Although *L. scariola* is a useless roadside weed in this country, it has long been cultivated in Europe as a medicine plant. The milky sap is collected, allowed to coagulate and then dried in the sun. The sun-dried extract is called "lactucarium" and was once listed as an official drug in the U.S.P. It was most often used for its sedative, pain-relieving and antispasmodic effects in place of opium, as it is much milder, will not damage the digestive system and has the advantage of being non-narcotic.

Lactucarium, and other extracts of wild lettuce, should not be used without competent supervision and must be discontinued after a short period of use.

Although most people think of garden lettuce *(Lactuca sativa)* as nothing more than a rather bland vehicle for salad dressing, it is also a useful medicine. It has the same properties as its wild relative but is much milder in its action. It is a mild diuretic, liver tonic, lowers the blood sugar, is calmative and anti-spasmodic. Since lettuce is always eaten before the bitter milk sap has a chance to develop, the garden

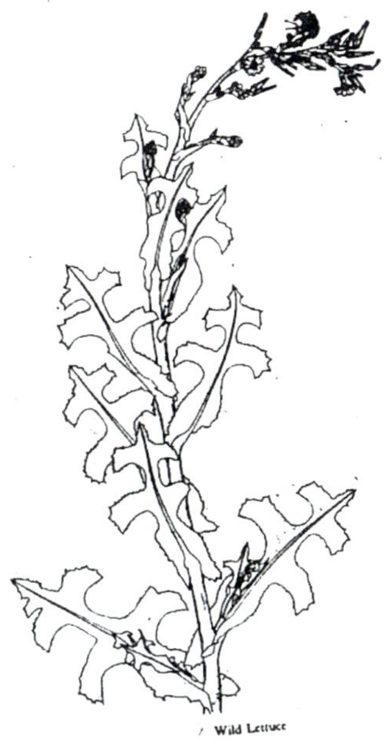

Wild Lettuce

variety must be allowed to "bolt" before it becomes pharmacologically active.

Lettuce tea can be made by infusing 3 ounces of the plant in 1 quart of water and drinking cupful at a time, 3-5 times daily. The same tea makes a soothing lotion for burns or a troubled complexion. Pulped lettuce leaves make a good poultice for wounds, burns or chest congestion. For chronic nervous and hepatic conditions, lettuce braised and eaten as a vegetable (3 plants daily) can be a valuable dietary supplement.

Lettuce may be mild, but it is potent. Augustus Caesar was cured of a liver complaint by eating lettuce, and was so grateful he erected an altar and statue in honor of this wonderful healing plant!

Marina Bokelman may be heard on HERB TALK, every Monday at 5 p.m. on KVMR, 89.5.

by Marina Bokelman

HERB TALK: Mugwort

That slender, unobtrusive silvery green plant growing in small communities along roadsides, creeksides, fence-rows and other waste areas at this time of year is Mugwort *(Artemisia vulgaris)*. The leaves of this perennial plant are easy to recognize, being green above and grey and downy beneath. The upper leaves are usually lanceolate while the lower are invariably lobed, resembling three-fingered hands. The flowers appear as round silvery balls along the panicled flower spike. When crushed, the foliage releases a strong pungent scent—a cross between sage and camphor. The taste? Bitter—like all the Artemisias.

The Artemisias take their name from Artemis, Greek goddess of healing and childbirth. And indeed, all the Artemisias are powerful healing plants, especially for women. A list of Artemisias reads like a roll-call of greats: Wormwood *(A absinthum)*, Southernwood *(A. abrotanum)*, Black Sagebrush *(A. tridentata*—so often used in Plains Indian sweat lodges), Moxa *(A. sinenis,* the down of which is rolled into cones for use in

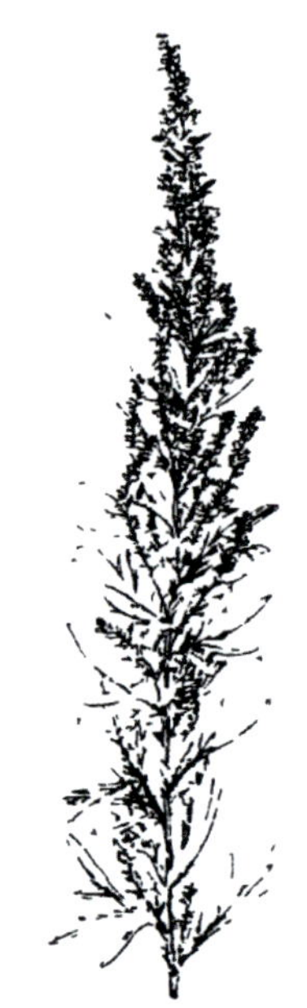

moxabustion, an Oriental healing technique associated with acupuncture), and Tarragon *(A. dracunculus)*.

Mugwort is tonic to the liver, gallbladder and spleen. In dilute doses it is an aid to the digestion and a remedy for nausea. It is also used as a diaphoretic, to break a cold at its onset.

The chief use of Mugwort, through the ages, has been as an emmenagogue—to normalize the menstrual flow. Hippocrates and Dioscorides praised it as a parturient, expediting labor and delivery.

Because emmenagogue herbs are so often misunderstood, let me point out here that Mugwort will not induce an abortion and should not be attempted for that purpose.

Mugwort, like its sister plant Wormwood, is an extremely powerful and potentially toxic plant. Large doses will cause purging and nervous symptoms.

A Mugwort tea made with 1 teaspoon of herb to 1 cup of water would be taken in mouthful doses, 2 or 3 times daily. Of the tincture, 5 drops would be a starting dose.

Externally, Mugwort has many uses. The poultice of fresh juice is soothing to poison oak rash, bruises and inflammatory swellings. Mugwort baths were once recommended for rheumatism and gout. Native Californians used Mugwort in their sweat lodges to treat rheumatism and arthritis. The affected limbs were bound with bundles of wet leaves (first bruised in a mortar) and then covered with earth while sweating.

Marina Bokelman may be heard on HERB TALK every Monday at 5 p.m. on KVMR, 89.5.

HERB TALK: The Almond

In Biblical times the Almond was reckoned as the best of all fruiting trees in the land of Canaan, and the delicate white blossoms, appearing in January, symbolized the dawn of creation. This member of the Rose Family (Rosaceae) is a native of West Asia and North Africa and was cultivated in Persia and China for several millenia before the birth of Christ. The Romans are responsible for introducing the Almond (like so many other useful plants) to Western Europe and the British Isles.

There are two varieties of Almond: the Sweet Almond (*Amygdalus communis* var. *dulcis)* and the Bitter Almond (*Amygdalus communis* var. *amara)*.

The Sweet Almond is highly nutritious. The nuts contain 20% protein and almost no starch, making them an ideal food for diabetics. They are excellent meat substitute, and Almond Milk (made by pounding the nuts with water) makes a good milk substitute for babies and invalids.

As a medicine plant the Sweet Almond is demulcent, both the oil and milk being used to soothe heartburn, gastric inflammation, constipation and hoarseness. These demulcent properties make Sweet Almond Oil an important ingredient in cosmetics, where it is often combined with Rosewater. The blossoms, leaves, bark and shells of the Sweet Almnd are used in folk medicine for their vermifuge, febrifuge, diuretic, hepatic and antitussive properties.

The Bitter Almond tells a different story. It contains the glucoside *amygdalin* which converts to Prussic (or hydrocyanic) acid. Prussic acid is one of the most toxic compounds found in nature, acting quickly to paralyze the central nervous system. It is found in all parts of the tree, especially the nut, which yields the deadly Oil of Bitter Almonds so favored by writers of murder mysteries.

Needless to say, the Bitter Almond should never be used internally. It can be used externally, however, as a poultice for the pain of neuralgia and migraine.

Marina Bokelman may be heard on HERB TALK, every Monday at 5 p.m. on KVMR, 89.5.

Apples

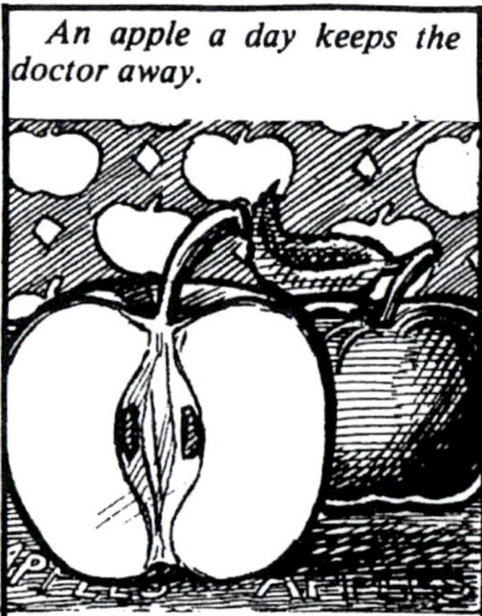

Now that Apple season is upon us. let's examine the truth in this old saying. The Apple *(Pyrus malus)* is a tasty and nourishing food, rich in vitamins, minerals and pectin, and, like its relatives in the Rosaceae Family (Roses, Strawberries, Raspberries, Blackberries and Almonds), it is also medicinal.

Apples contain malic, oxalic and tartaric acids and are tonic to the liver and to the digestive and urinary systems. Apples are also cooling and cleansing to the blood—they eliminate uric acid from the system, making them useful for gout and rheumatism. In Normandy, where unsweetened cider is the daily beverage, urinary stone is virtually unknown. And experiments have shown that typhoid bacilli do not live long in fresh apple juice.

An Apple a day in the morning will cleanse the body of waste products of the previous day; an Apple a day at night is a remedy for constipation (as are stewed Apples). Grated Apples (slightly unripe) are a remedy for diarrhea and bilious indigestion. The old-fashioned practice of serving applesauce with pork or goose and of eating Apples with cheese is a healthy one—the Apples assist the digestion in handling these rich fatty foods. A raw Apple also cleanses the teeth.

Needless to say, fresh ripe Apples plucked from unsprayed trees make the best medicine. You cannot assume that the Apples you buy at the store have any value at all after commercial cultivation, spraying and cold storage.

The bark of the Apple tree is a bitter tonic, stimulant and febrifuge, and has been used as a substitute for quinine in intermittent and bilious fevers. A decoction of Apple bark also acts to constrict the blood vessels. The leaves, buds and blossoms of the Apple are diuretic and can be used for urinary inflammations and stone. The peel of **unsprayed** Apples may be dried (instead of discarding them when you make jelly) and made into a tea for rheumatic ailments.

In mythology, Apples are associated with immortality. Avalon, the mysterious island where King Arthur sleeps until his people again need him, means "Apple Orchards." In the Druidic tradition of Ireland, the Apple is one of the seven Chieftain Trees and severe penalties fell on the person who cut one down.

In England, the old custom of wassailing the Apple trees still survives in some places. On Old 12th Night (January 17) the family takes offerings of bread and cider into the orchard and toasts the best bearing trees:

Here's to thee, old apple tree!
Whence thou may'st bud, and whence thou may'st blow:
Hats full! Caps full!
Bushel, bushel-bags full!
And my pockets full too! Huzza!

The Wassail Bowl contained roasted apples floating in hot spiced cider, wine or ale, and it was considered good luck to eat one of these apples. This must be the origin of our bobbing for apples on Halloween (which the Celts called the Feast of Apple-Gathering!).

Marina Bokelman

HERBS AS FOOD & MEDICINE

Let thy kitchen be thy apothecary and let foods be thy medicine.

—Hippocratus

A Medicine Plant (we usually call it an Herb, whether or not it is technically herbaceous) is one that is able to correct a condition of ill health. A Food Plant (we usually call it a vegetable, fruit, nut or grain) is one that is able to sustain both life and health. Some Medicine Plants, because of their ghastly taste (Goldenseal), powerful and specific action (Cascara Sagrada) or toxic side effects in large amounts (Wormwood), are never used for food. Many of the Food Plants, however, are very useful medicines.

Let's take a look at Cabbage. It can be prepared as a medicine for various conditions — the juice as an ulcer remedy or to expel worms, and a poultice of the leaves as a treatment for leg ulcers or lumbago. Cabbage can also be *eaten* as a therapeutic food to correct various conditions of ill health, especially problems of the digestive or respiratory systems.

Time is a factor, of course. One bowl of Cabbage soup will not cure your chronic bronchitis. It has taken the body many years to reach its condition of ill health and it will take many months to remedy that condition. Added to the diet in quantity, however, Cabbage (and many other therapeutic foods) can assist the body in its healing process. Or, you can eat Cabbage as preventive medicine, to strengthen and protect your body.

Wintertime, with its attendant sore throats and respiratory problems, is an ideal time to feature Cabbage. Since there is a limit to the amount of Cole Slaw anyone can eat, I offer a few of my favorite ways of eating Cabbage.

Cabbage Salad I - Finely shred Green Cabbage and toss with unrefined Corn oil (dark in color and rich in flavor) and a touch of Cumin (digestive and anti-flatulent), toasted lightly and crushed in a mortar and pestle.

Cabbage Salad II - Finely shred Red Cabbage, add chopped Watercress (antiseptic) and sliced Mushrooms. Toss with Oriental-style Sesame oil and Soy sauce.

Marina Bokelman

HERB TALK:

Horseradish

By Marina Bokelman

The humble Horseradish *(Cochlearia armoracia)* is a much neglected medicinal herb. Cultivated since earliest times, it was universally recognized as medicine long before its use as a condiment. It is so useful, prolific and easily grown that no home medicine chest should be without it.

When the fresh root is bruised, the glucoside *sinigrin* and the enzyme *myrosin* (found in separate plant cells) are allowed to interact, forming the volatile oil *allyl*. It is allyl that gives Horseradish its pungent aroma and hot biting taste. It is also the major medicinal ingredient.

Horseradish is primarily a stimulant: internally it stimulates a sluggish liver and bowel; externally it stimulates local circulation to promote healing and relieve pain and stiffness of rheumatism, gout, sciatica, neuralgia and congested conditions of the lungs, liver and kidneys. To make a Horseradish Poultice: grate the fresh root and place between two soft cottom cloths, binding over the affected part. Remove when the skin turns pink or a burning sensation is felt.

Horseradish is also diuretic, antiseptic, diaphoretic (promotes cleansing through perspiration) and vermifuge (expels worms). As a stomachic it assists in complete digestion of rich protein foods (hence its use as a condiment for oily fish and heavy meats), and cleanses the intestinal tract of the waste products of faulty digestion.

One of the best home uses of Horseradish is as a syrup for use as an expectorant (breaking up of mucous and congestion in the respiratory system) in cases of coughs, colds, hoarseness and sinus. Here are two recipes for Horseradish Syrup. **Quick:** grate 1-3 tsp. fresh root into ½ cup hot water, cover and let steep two hours. Add enough honey to make a thin syrup. **Not So Quick:** grate 2 ounces fresh root into 1 pint natural apple cider vinegar, cover and let steep 36 hours. Strain and add enough honey or pure vegetable glycerin to make a thin syrup. Start with 1 tsp. (less for children) three times daily or as needed.

More hardy individuals may wish to try Horseradish Slurry: grate fresh root and add enough fresh lemon juice or apple cider vinegar to make a thick sauce. Start with ¼ tsp. and hold in the mouth until all fumes have evaporated before swallowing. You will feel the mucous start to break loose at once. The Slurry should be refrigerated and made fresh every two days.

Like Black Mustardseed (which also contains allyl), large doses of Horseradish are emetic. Also, prolonged inhalation of the volatile oil or prolonged contact with the skin may cause irritation and burning.

Marina Bokelman can be heard with HERB TALK at its NEW time every Wednesday at 5 p.m. on KVMR 89.5

Cabbage

It is with good reason that the Walrus linked Cabbages with Kings as a topic worthy of discussion. The common garden Cabbage *(Brassica olearacea* var. *capitata)* has long been hailed as a healer — from Chryssipus the Greek (who said "The man who eats **Cabbage every day will** never have any medical problems") to French naturopaths who call it "the doctor of the poor." In Europe, where nutritional and herbal therapies are much more common, many serious and chronic conditions of the lungs, stomach, liver and bladder are treated with a diet of Cabbage (juice, salad, soup, steamed), followed for a period of months.

Freshly extracted Cabbage juice is anteseptic, decongestive and rich in **Vitamin U (soothing to the** mucosa), and is therefore useful for tonsillitis, hoarseness (made into a syrup with equal parts honey), and inflammations of the digestive tract, including ulcers. Cabbage juice is also a vermifuge.

As a poultice plant Cabbage should be part of **everyone's home, remedy** repetoire. It has the ability to draw toxins out of the body and then stimulate healing. Cuts, bites, stings, swellings, burns, bruises and infected wounds may be treated by this method. To make a Cabbage poultice, first remove the tough midrib. You may then crush the leaves with a rolling pin and bind several layers to the affected area, **or pound them into a pulp with mortar and pestle before binding into place. For very** you may wish to blanch the leaves for a few minutes in boiling water, making them soft and tender.

Cabbages poultices have even been used for such serious and/or chronic conditions as abscesses, animal bites, eczema, leg ulcers, gangrene, rheumatism, gout, lumbago, neuralgia and sciatica. With such serious conditions, a *healing crisis* may occur. Such flare-up of **symptoms is caused by the body suddenly being stimulated into the activity of throwing off toxins and healing itself. If such a flare-up occurs, soothe the affected area with olive oil and** resume the Cabbage treatment after a day or two, using shorter applications.

Meanwhile, even if you are not sick, Cabbage can be enjoyed as a highly nutritious food, rich in the stress vitamins and minerals (C, B6, calcium, magnesium), sulphur, iron, copper and iodine. People with delicate digestion should try cabbage cooked with caraway, cumin or dill (all carminatives!) or as naturally fermented sauerkraut.

Sauerkraut - Finely shred Green Cabbage (or chop finely in a wooden bowl) and pack into quart jars, leaving 1½ inches of headroom. To each quart add 1 tsp non-iodized salt and fill with pure water. Screw on canning lids *loosely* and let stand for a few days until fermentation is complete. Add more water if necessary and tighten lids — there is no need to process. The lactic acid in naturally fermented Sauerkraut will cleanse the digestive tract from top to bottom and help restore proper functioning of the digestive system.

And don't forget Cabbage Soup!

HERB TALK:

Herbal Antiseptics—Myrrh

Now that winter is here with a new crop of colds and flu, it is time to look at the antiseptic *(anti*-against, *septic*-infected, toxic) herbs. Some herbal antiseptics, like Goldenseal and Garlic, have bacteriostatic properties, inhibiting the growth of bacteria. Others, such as Echinacea and Myrrh, help the body mobilize its own resources to fight off infection and eliminate toxins.

Myrrh *(Commiphora myrrha)* is a large woody shrub native to the Middle East where it was been used for over 4,000 years as an ingredient in perfumes, oils and incense (used for fumigation as well as ritual). In Biblical times, Myrrh, along with Francincense and other herbs and spices, was valued equal to gold and precious gems.

The medicinal portion of the plant is the resin, which is collected from fissures in the bark and allowed to harden. This is then powdered and sold as Gum Myrrh.

Taken internally, Myrrh actually increases the white blood count, significantly enhancing the body's ability to fight off bacterial infections. It stimulates circulation by quickening heart action and acts as an expectorant, ueful in chronic catarrh. It is eliminated by the body through the bronchial and genitourinary membranes and has a decongestive and disinfecting effect on them.

Myrrh is also an astringent and stimulating healer for damaged body tissues. The powdered gum may be sprinkled directly onto fresh wounds to stop bleeding and prevent infection. Because of these qualities and its specific tonic effect on the mucous membranes, Myrrh makes a useful gargle for problems of the throat and mouth. The powder, mixed with equal parts of Goldenseal root powder, can be brushed into the gums in cases of pyorrhea.

Myrrh is best taken in tincture form, 10 to 30 drops in a glass of water as needed. For an infusion, use ½ tsp. of the powdered gum to 1 cup of boiling water and take in 1 Tb. doses 3 to 6 times daily. Large doses of Myrrh cause vomiting and purging and may over-stimulate the heart.

HERB TALK:

HOLLY & IVY

*Christmastide
Comes in like a bride
With Holly and Ivy clad*

Christmas is here and it is time to deck the halls with wreaths of Holly *(Ilex aquifolium)* and Ivy *(Hedera helix)*. The two plants—tree and vine, prickly and smooth, red-berried and white-berried — make an interesting contrast.

The custom of decorating the dwelling with greenery in midwinter comes to us courtesy of the Romans (who used evergreen boughs as house decorations during Saturnalia) and the Druids (who brought in evergreens to make winter homes for forest spirits). Because the birth of Christ occurs at the same time of year as a number of important pagan ceremonies, the Nativity is now associated with some of the old practices.

The Holly Tree has particularly associated itself with Christian legend. Also called *Holy Tree* and *Christ's Thorn*, the plant is said to have sprung up from Christ's footprints.

Holly leaves are the medicinal part of the plant, being diaphoretic and expectorant. The tea is also used as a tonic febrifuge for intermittent fevers and inflammation of the joints. A brew of 1-2 Tb of the leaves to 1 cup of water would be a standard dose. Leaves of another species *(Ilex paraguayensis)* are known to us as the familiar tea substitute — Yerba Mate.

The **berries** of the Holly Tree are to be avoided, being violently emetic and purgative, even in small doses. They are especially dangerous to children.

Common English Ivy was once used by Dionysian revelers as a crown in honor of the God. Later, English taverns would display the sign of the Ivy Bush to advertise the quality of the spirits within. Hence: "Good wine needs no bush."

Although Ivy has been used medicinally by experienced herbalists for various dropsical and bilious complaints, this herb can be quite toxic when incorrectly used. Overdose causes vomiting, purging and serious disturbances of the stomach, blood pressure and nerves.

However, Ivy can be used **externally** in the form of a fomentation or poultice to relieve the pain of swollen joints and glands (mumps). For an earache or toothache, a cotton cloth can be soaked in a brew of Ivy leaves and applied hot to the outside of the head or jaw. Ivy extracts are currently used in European spas as part of a treatment to reduce cellulite.

So, for Good Medicine and Good Cheer

*Sing holly, sing ivy
Sing ivy, sing holly
A drop just to drink
It would cure melancholy*
By Marina Bokelman

HEALTH TALK/HERB TALK

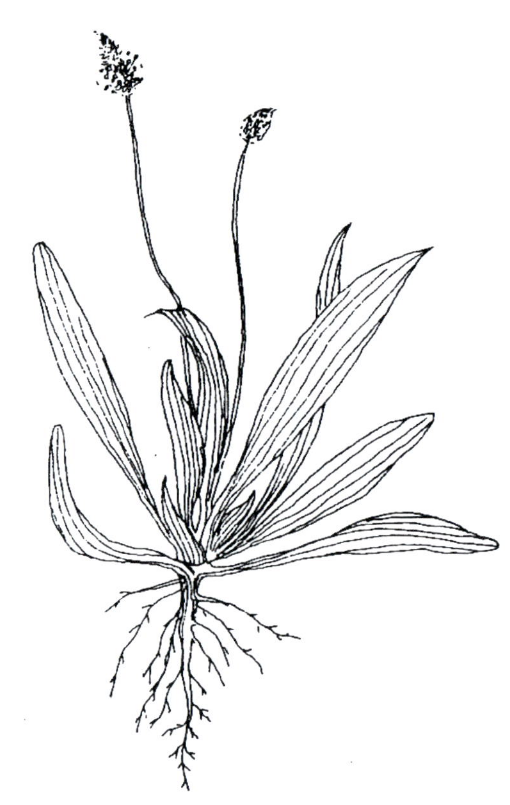

89.5 FM KVMR 89.5 FM KVMR 89.5 FM KVMR

8 Airnotes — Fall 1984

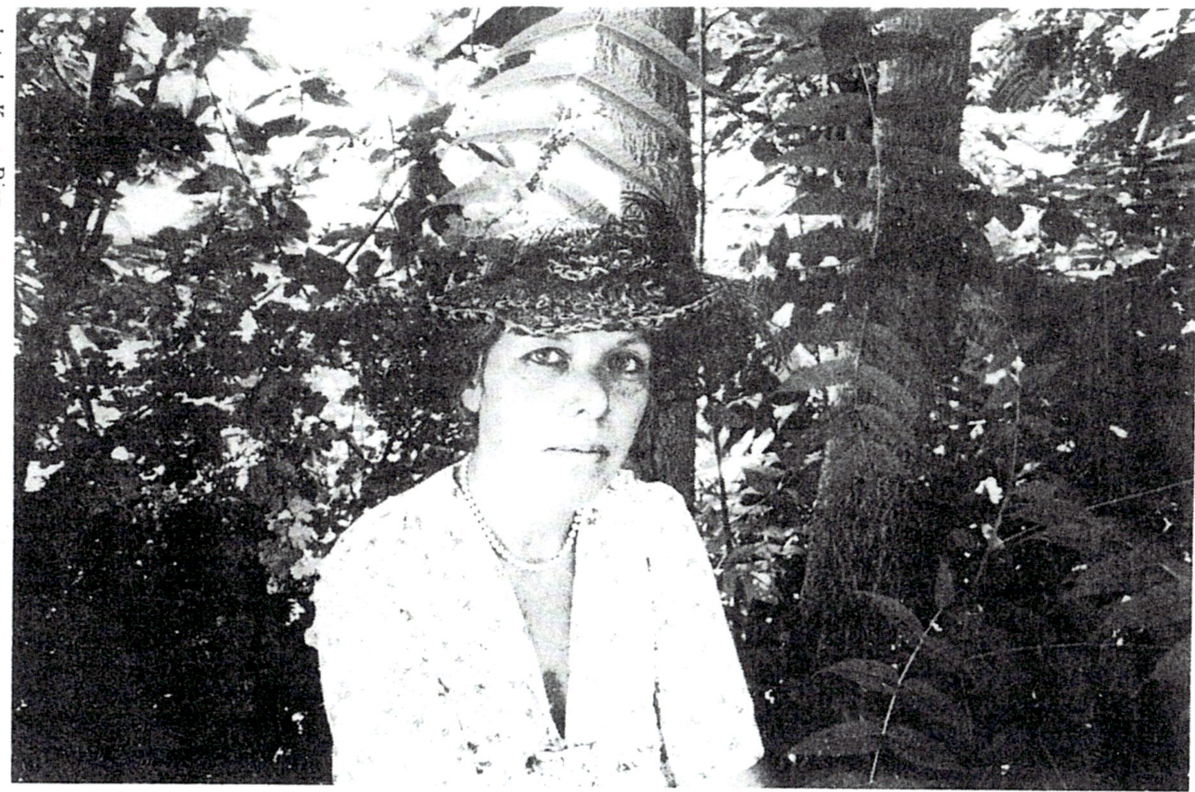

MARINA BOKLEMAN

HEALTH TALK/HERB TALK

The following is a condensed excerpt from the July 16th broadcast of "Health Talk" during which Jeff Kane interviewed herbologist Marina Bokelman. Marina has been working with herbs since 1969. She gives classes and consultations, and is the founder of Medicine Flower, a small company dedicated to making traditional herbal remedies. She can be heard every Wednesday at 5:00 p.m. on "Herb Talk", a 15-minute information segment of "Music Magazine", during which she discusses the properties and purposes of various herbs.

Jeff Kane is an M.D. He currently teaches Iyengar-style yoga and gives workshops in pain management. His show, "Health Talk", is a call-in/interview program devoted to discussion of health issues, and can be heard every Monday from 7:00 to 8:00 p.m.

J: I'm aware that you have skills that you could easily be making a living at, but you've chosen herbalism. How do you know it's your calling?

M: Because I just keep doing it; I can't help it.

J: How did you first hear from inside that herbs are what you're supposed to do?

M: I first heard the message when I was a child but I didn't understand it. I actually remember the first time somebody told me a plant was good for something. For a long time I picked up information without knowing why. Then when I was grown I had a personal health crisis and suddenly everything I had learned became important. At that point I was on the path — working with herbs in a focused way for myself and for others.

J: I was trained as an M.D. in the theory of the Magic Bullet — that each disease is caused by a single micro-organism, and if you find the specific chemical that will kill it, you will cure the disease.

M: I never think about killing germs specifically. If you come to me with a terribly sore throat, there are herbal protocols I can follow which are highly effective for any infectious condition, which will mobilize your immune system, cleanse your bloodstream and ease your symptoms. Chances are you'll be better in the same time it would have taken to send out a throat culture to find the exact name of the germ.

J: If you ask me how penicillin works I'll give you a biochemical explanation. What's your explanation for how herbs work?

M: You can also explain herbs biochemically because they have a biochemical action. I don't have that training. I use a more old-fashioned set of metaphors — I talk about cleansing and toning and about the affinities that herbs have for certain organs or systems. The important thing is not the language you use but the depth of understanding and experience you bring to your practice.

J: What causes disease? I don't suppose you can say disease is a shortage of herbs any more than insanity is a shortage of Thorazine.

M: Herbs have a very different relationship to us than drugs like thorazine. I call an herb, a medicine plant, any plant that will promote, maintain or restore health. This gives us a spectrum ranging from plants we call "food" to plants we call "medicine"— all a food plant is is a palatable and benign medicine. Plants like Apples or Cabbage can keep you healthy when you eat them as foods, but they can also be used as medicine when health becomes unbalanced. A lot of plants we think of as culinary herbs — Rosemary, Thyme, Sage, Garlic — are

extremely powerful medicines. Most people just don't think of them that way. Now if health becomes seriously unbalanced, you may have to use an herb that has an unpleasant taste, like Goldenseal or Gentian, or an herb with extremely powerful action, like Poke. In the days before antibiotics, purging herbs saved lives. So in a way, yes, disease *is* an absence of herbs. Because it means you're not using healing plants in your life in the right way. This can be everything from diet to tonic adjustments you can make on a daily basis to simple remedial protocols using safe and accessible herbs like Echinacea or Mullein. In Europe, many people still routinely drink herb teas. They are a pleasant beverage, but there is the knowledge that if you tend to have poor circulation or heart trouble runs in the family, you'll take Rosemary or Hawthorn. If you're a nervous kind of person, maybe you'll choose Linden blossoms or Lemon Balm for your daily tea. If you incorporate these healing plants into your life, it's a way to be well. And a beautiful and harmonious way to be in the world.

J: What you're talking about here is medicine that is free, that is pleasant and congenial.

M: A lot of these plants have been following our footsteps from the beginning of the human race, trying to get our attention, saying "Use me!" The minute you clear some land, what do you get? Dandelion, Plantain, Yellow Dock, Chickweed, Shepard's Purse, Thistles. These are all healing plants but we call them "weeds."

J: I talk to different practitioners who use different modalities and they all work. Is the common denominator the change in consciousness of the person who is sick?

M: There has to be a change in consciousness for true healing to occur. All the placebo effect is is the activation of the person's inner ability to heal himself. I believe that all healers should strive to activate the placebo effect. But I also believe that herbs have an action beyond the placebo effect. Actually, I'm glad there are so many ways for people to be healed. It would be terrible if there were only one way of healing and only one group of people in charge of it.

(The above is a condensed excerpt from "HealthTalk, 7/16/84)

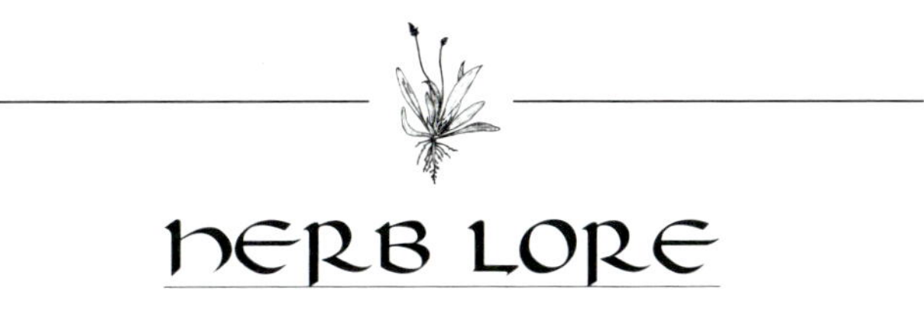

ḢERB LORE

ABOUT THE RIDDLES, STORIES AND SONGS

Riddles, stories and songs are all forms of what is called *folklore*, or "wisdom of the people". These forms of lore are not just for entertainment in traditional cultures lacking television and other forms of commercially produced entertainment. They are vehicles for teaching as well. They have a marvelous ability to hold, preserve and transmit information from one generation to the next.

I was lucky. I grew up in a family where songs, stories, riddles, fables, circular stories and every other kind of lore, were a part of everyday life. My parents and maternal grandmother sang songs from their respective traditions and I learned early and eagerly. My mother especially was a fountain of folk lore. Perhaps it is not surprising that when I went to university at UCLA, my undergraduate degree was in Cultural Anthropology, and my Master's degree was in Folklore & Mythology.

RIDDLES

These two riddles I learned from a wonderful boxed set of records issued by the Archive of Folk Song, Library of Congress, called *The Hammons Family: A Study of a West Virginia Family's Traditions*. In the Hammons family, riddling was one way in which the younger generation was educated. Maggie Hammons relates that her father used to take all ten children out walking in the deep woods. He would stop suddenly and give out with: "Crooked like a rainbow, teeth like a cat/You can guess all night but you can't guess that." All the children would look around, analyzing their habitat and everything growing in it until one of them would get it. She said her father would not move on until someone got the answer or he instructed them in the meaning of the riddle. It was a brilliant teaching technique. Once I heard these riddles, I never forgot them.

RIDDLE #1

Crooked like a rainbow
Teeth like a cat
You can guess all night
But you can't guess that

What am I?

RIDDLE #2

White I am
      But snow I ain't
Green I am
      But grass I ain't
Red I am
      But blood I ain't
Black I am
      But coal I ain't

What am I?

ANSWER #1

I am **Greenbriar** or **Cat Briar**

My canes arch like a rainbow
My thorns bite like a cat

ANSWER #2

I am **Blackberry**

My blossoms are as white as newest snow
My early fruits are hard and green as grass
My half-ripe berries turn to red like blood
My sweetest, ripest fruits are black as coal

STORIES

These two stories are of the type called "etiological tales" or "origin stories". They explain why something is the way it is—how it came to be a certain way. Some of us grew up with Rudyard Kipling's wonderful *Just So Stories*: "How the Leopard Got Its Spots", "How the Elephant Got Its Trunk", "How the Camel Got Its Hump", and so forth.

I heard "The Old Man's Winter Gloves" as an untitled outline by storyteller Steve Sanfield on San Juan Ridge where I moved in 1979. The story filled itself in based on my earlier experiences in North Carolina. The herbal knowledge embedded in this tale will help you identify an important medicine plant (I'm not going to give this one away).

"How Milk Thistle and Deer Brought Back Fire" came to me while I was harvesting Milk Thistle seeds in clothing inappropriate for the job—a suit of armor would have been better than the gauze blouse, thin cotton skirt and sandals I was wearing. As I pressed my body deeper and deeper into the enormous milk thistle plants in order to harvest the seeds, the razor sharp edges of the leaves with their hard thorny prickles pierced my clothing and skin. I thought of the experience as an herbalist's Sun Dance.

As I stood in the hot sun, harvesting seeds from this valuable liver regenerative plant, the story came to me, and as it came I memorized it.

The story is a version of the universal tale about the theft of fire, but set in the pattern of a California Native creation tale. And so we have Coyote and Silver Fox and Turtle as Earth Diver. But embedded in this story is a teaching about which medicine plants have hollow stalks--because the living coal of stolen fire had to be sealed up and carried back in a receptacle that would hold it. It also explains something about Deer's abilities.

To get a sense of California Indian culture and storytelling, take a look at Jaime de Angulo's *Indian Tales* and *Indians in Overalls*. For many more tales try *Californian Indian Nights Entertainments* compiled by Edward W. Gifford and Gwendoline Harris Block.

THE OLD MAN'S WINTER GLOVES

A long time ago, at the head of the holler, there lived an old man and an old woman. They lived very well, between what they raised in the garden and what they gathered in the woods, and the old man was still a good hand at hunting and fishing. They had a few chickens for the eggs, of course, and a hog to fatten for winter.

One winter the old man came to the old woman and said, "Honey, the older I get, the colder my hands get. "Do you think you could knit me a pair of warm winter gloves?"

The old woman said, "Well, I never have knit a pair of gloves in my life, but I love you, and I'll try."

The very day the old man whittled his wife a set of wooden knitting pins. The next day the old woman traded a dozen eggs for some woolen yarn from a spinning woman down the road. Then she commenced to knitting.

The first pair of gloves the old woman made looked like this. [Show thumb and fingers all held close together] The old man tried them on. "Honey," he said, "these are mighty soft and warm, but I won't be able to get a grip on the axe handle with my thumb and fingers bunched up together like this." So, the old woman took the gloves and threw them out back on a little bush.

The next pair of gloves the old woman made looked like this. [Show thumb separate, the rest of the fingers close together] The old man put them on and went outside to do his chores. After a while he came back in and said, "Honey, these are dandy for chopping wood, but I can't manage the plow hitch or the latch on the gate without my forefinger loose." So, the old woman took the gloves and threw them out back on the little bush.

The third pair of gloves the old woman made looked like this [Show thumb separate, forefinger separate, the rest of the fingers held close together] The old man put them on and went about his business. In the evening he came back in and said to his wife, "Honey, these are the best yet, but there are still some chores I can't do without the use of all my fingers." So the old woman took the gloves and threw them out back on the little bush.

Well, the last pair of gloves the old woman made looked like this. [Show thumb and all fingers spread wide apart] The old man tried them on and said he was well pleased with his warm winter gloves. The old woman said she was well satisfied with her handiwork, and put the knitting pins away.

The last I heard, the old man and the old woman were still living there at the head of the holler and doing mighty well.

And that little bush out in the back? Why that became the Sassafras!!

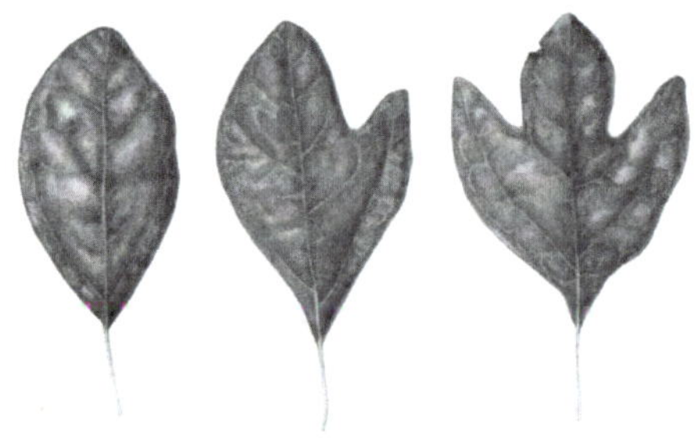

HOW DEER AND MILK THISTLE BROUGHT BACK FIRE

All stories begin with the Creation

I guess you heard about how Creator made the world from his breath and from the sweat and dirt he rubbed from his body. Then he Dreamed—and the spark of life came into the world through the crack the Dreaming made. Then Creator gave the world to Coyote and Silver Fox and the rest of them so they could make the world good. This they did, putting the mountains and rivers in their places, hanging the clouds in the heavens, and placing stars and stones for guidance.

Things were good for a long time. Then anger came into the world. Each one was afraid that there was not enough goodness for all. So there was envy and greed and anger, and the world burned. It burned. It burned for a long time. Smoke covered the sky and the sun could no longer be seen.

Then the people prayed for healing and it began to rain. First a little, and then so much that the waters ran over the surface of the earth. Then all the waters ran together until there was nothing but water everywhere.

For a long time this continued. Then the people began to talk among themselves. Who will dive down to the bottom of the waters and bring back some earth with which to make the world again. I guess you heard how it was Turtle, after all the others failed, who dove to the very bottom of the waters and brought back a fist full of mud gripped in her little claws.

From this handful of earth they made the world again.

At first everything was good. It was summertime, and there were berries and wild fruits in abundance. But soon the days shortened and the nights turned cold. People began to miss their warm, cozy fires. All had been lost in the great flood. Without fire in the hearth, there was no warmth or cheer in the long, cold nights. There was no way to cook food, and medicines could not be made. Worst of all, there was no circle of light and warmth around which to gather in the long winter nights to hear the songs and stories of the Elders.

So people got to talking. Someone heard that the people in the South had gotten fire from a Fire Mountain they had down there. A delegation of Elders was chosen to speak for the people and ask for the gift of fire. Four times they asked. Four times they were refused.

Again the people gathered to talk. "Who will steal fire," they asked, "so the people may live in comfort and harmony again?" "I will," said Cricket. "I am so little and light, no one will see me. I will carry a hollow stalk of Fennel to keep the fire in."

Next day Cricket set off and soon came to the Fire Mountain. After dark he crept in and took a living coal, sealing it up in the hollow stalk of Fennel. He hadn't gone too far towards home when he became tired and decided to rest. Well, you know how Crickets are—they cannot resist making music. Cricket scraped away at his fiddle and the Fire Mountain people heard him. They followed the sound, and finding Cricket, they beat him up and took their fire back.

The next volunteer was Mouse. "I am very quiet," she said, "no one will hear me. I will take a hollow stick of Elder to keep the fire in."

So Mouse set off, and soon came to the Fire Mountain. She crept in after dark, took a living coal and sealed it up in the hollow stick of Elder. She hadn't gone far towards home when she became sleepy and decided to rest. But you know how timid Mice are. She had to make herself a tiny fire, just for cheer. But the Fire Mountain people saw the light and followed it. Finding Mouse, they beat her up and took their fire back.

No one knew what to do. Then a voice spoke up from the back. It was Milk Thistle, a small, nondescript prickley thistle growing at the edge of the meadow, too shy to come into the open. "I will get the fire," said Milk Thistle. "They will not dare to grasp me and take back the fire. But someone must carry me." Different ones tried, but no one could hold the Milk Thistle, the edges of her leaves were so sharp. Deer finally came forward. "I will carry you," she said. "My mouth is tender, but

I am not afraid. I will do this as a Giveaway for the People."

The next day, Milk Thistle and Deer set off, and soon came to the Fire Mountain. After dark, they crept down, took a living coal, and sealed it within the hollow stem of the Milk Thistle. As Deer was light of foot and had great stamina, they brought the fire back without mishap. Once again there was light and warmth and cheer, and all the People were glad.

The people held a great ceremony for Milk Thistle and Deer. Milk Thistle they honored with offerings of pollen, which became the white blotches and streaks you see on the leaves of the Milk Thistle today. She was given the right to stand tall and proud in the center of the meadow, crowned in purple, giving healing and light to all. And the Deer, well Deer was given the gift to be able to eat anything prickley or thorny. Especially your rose bushes!!

SONGS

"**The Bitter Withy**" is one of my favorite ballads. The story is from the Folk Apocrypha, meaning stories about the life of Jesus not found in the Bible.

This ballad tells the story of an immature shaman, an individual with great power who is still a child, with the emotions and actions of a child, who has not yet learned how to use power responsibly. Yes, children were sometimes "switched" with the thin, flexible Willow withies when they were naughty. But the last verse makes this song into an etiological tale because it explains why the taste of this medicine plant is so exceedingly bitter and why the wood rots so easily. As an herbalist, I find a deeper meaning. The salicin found in Willow bark (from which aspirin was derived) can relieve pain, in this case the pain of being switched with a handful of willow twigs.

"**The Simpler's Alphabet**" is one of my "air songs", as my friend, blues man Robert Pete Williams called the songs that came to him "out of the air". I moved to Nevada County in 1979 and in the first two years worked hard to establish myself as an herbal healer. I was teaching a two weekend herb skills workshop (making infusions, decoctions, poultices, salves, fomentations, tinctures, glycerites and more).

This meant driving the South Fork of the Yuba River Canyon two times a day for two weekends for a total of eight, lovely 50 minute drives, with a hillside of *Sticky Monkey Flower* on the left as you came to the bottom of the grade and a nice patch of *Mugwort* on the

River side as you started to climb out.

As each line of the song came in, I memorized it, and then practiced singing the whole verse until I was confident I would remember it.

Certain songs of sailors and lumberjacks are called "occupational folksongs." **The Alphabet Song** of each of these professions is meant to teach the beginner the tools of his trade.

The sailors sing:
A is for Anchor, that we all do know
and then go on to *B is for Bowline*, one of the knots a sailor's life depends upon.

Lumberjacks sing:
A is for Axe, that we all do know
And so on. Both are sung to the same tune and end with the same verse:

W, X, Y, Z makes rhyming go wrong
And now I have come to the end of my song

When I sang *The Simplers' Alphabet* at Breitenbush Herbal Gathering where I was teaching that year, a young, earnest herb student suggested that I could have gone on with *Wormwood, Xanthoxylum (Prickley Ash Bark)* and *Yarrow*, and was perplexed when I replied that it was *traditional* for the singer to end the song in that way.

BITTER WITHY

A high holiday and a bright holiday
Small hail from the sky did fall
Our Savior asked his Mother dear
If he might go play at ball

"At ball, at ball, my own dear son
'Twas time that you were gone
But don't let me hear of any mischief
At night when you come home"

So up the hill and down the hill
Our sweet young Savior run
Until he met three rich young lords
"Good morning" to each one

"Good morn", "good morn", "good morn"
    said they
"Good morning" then said he
"Now which of you three rich young lords
Will play at ball with me?"

"We are all lords and ladies sons
Born in a bower and hall
And you are nothing but a poor maid's child
Born in an ox's stall"

Then Jesus turned him round about
He did neither laugh nor smile
But the tears come a trickling down his cheeks
Like water from the sky

So he built him a bridge of the beams of the
    sun
And over the water ran he
The rich young lords chased after him
And drowned they were all three

Then up the hill and down the hill
Three rich young mothers run
Saying "Mary mild fetch home your child
For ours he's drowned each one"

So Mary mild fetched home her child
And laid him across her knee
And with a handful of Willow twigs
She gave him lashes three

"Ah bitter Withy, ah bitter Withy
And the Willow it doth smart
And the Willow shall be the very first tree
To perish at the heart"

*— I learned this song from the singing of
    A. L. Lloyd, one of the best ballad singers in
    the British Isles.*

THE SIMPLER'S ALPHABET SHEET MUSIC

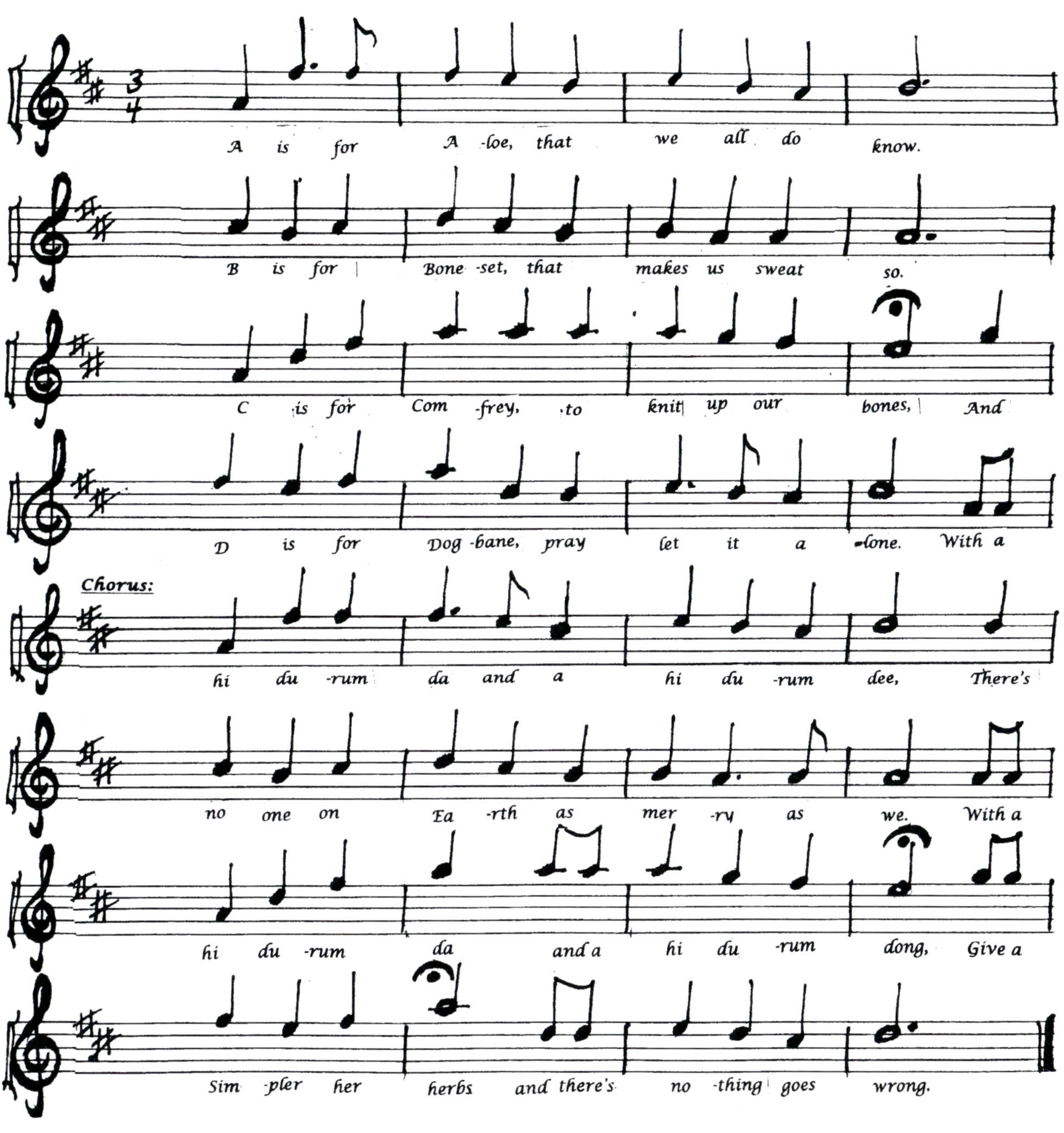

THE SIMPLER'S ALPHABET

	A is for	A-loe, that	we all do	know.
	B is for	Bone-set, that	makes us sweat	so.
	C is for	Com-frey, to	knit up our	bones,
And	D is for	Dog-bane, pray	let it	alone.

Chorus:

With a.	hi du-rum	da and a	hi du-rum	dee,
There's	no one on	Ea-rth as	mer-ry as	we.
With a	hi du-rum	da and a	hi du-rum	dong,
Give a	Sim-pler her	herbs and there's	no-thing goes	wrong.

	E"s E-chi	-na-cea, or	Samp-son Snake	Root.
	Fen-nel gives	com-fort when	beans make us	toot.
	Deep, war-ming Gin-ger drives	out cold and	damp,
And	H is for	Haw Bark, which	eas-es a	cramp.

(chorus)

	Tried and true	bl-ue is	In-di-go's	worth.
	Ja-lap will	purge you like	no-thing on	Earth.
	K's for the	Kiss of the	rain on the	ground,
And	L is for	Love, which makes	heal-ing a	-bound.

(chorus)

	M is for	Mug-wort, to	o-pen our	dreams.
	N is for	No-thing that	is as it	seems.
	O is for	On-ion, to	poul-tice our	chest,
And re	-mem-ber with	Poke Root, small	dos-age is	best.

(chorus)

	Queen of the	Mea-dow gives	gra-vel a	start.
	Rosemary	cir-cu-lates	Love through the	heart.
	S is for	Sage, which we	all hope to	be,
And	Thy-mus Vul	-ga-ris will	plea-sure your	bees.

(chorus)

	U is for	Un-guent to	heal up our	sores.
	V is for	Vio-let, that	blooms when it	thaws.
	W,X,Y,	-Z makes the	rhym-ing go	wrong,
And	now I have	come to the	end of my	song.

Chorus:

With a.	hi du-rum	da and a	hi du-rum	dee,
There's	no one on	Ea-rth as	mer-ry as	we.
With a	hi du-rum	da and a	hi du-rum	dong,
Give a	Sim-pler her	herbs and there's	no-thing goes	wrong.

THE SIMPLER'S ALPHABET

A is for **Aloe** that we all do know
B is for **Boneset** that makes us sweat so
C is for **Comfrey** to knit up our bones
And **D** is for **Dog Bane**, pray let it alone

Cho: With a hi durum dah, and a hi durum dee
            There's no one on earth as merry as we
      With a hi durum dah and a hi durum dong
            Give a Simpler her herbs and there's nothing goes wrong

E's **Echinacea** or Samson Snake Root
F is for **Fennel** when beans make us toot
Deep warming **Ginger** drives out cold and damp
And **H** is for **Haw Bark** that eases a cramp

Tried and true blue is **Indigo**'s worth
Jalap will purge you like nothing on earth
K's for the **Kiss** of the rain on the ground
And **L** is for **Love** that makes healing abound

M is for **Mugwort** to open our dreams
N is for **Nothing** that is as it seems
O is for **Onion** to poultice our chest
And remember with **Poke Root** small dosage is best

Queen of the Meadow gives gravel a start
Rosemary circulates love through the heart
S is for **Sage** which we all hope to be
And **Thymus vulgaris** will pleasure your bees

U is for **Unguent** to heal up our sores
V is for **Violet** that blooms when it thaws
W X Y Z makes rhyming go wrong
And now I have come to the end of my song

— Driving the River Canyon, South Fork of the Yuba, 1983

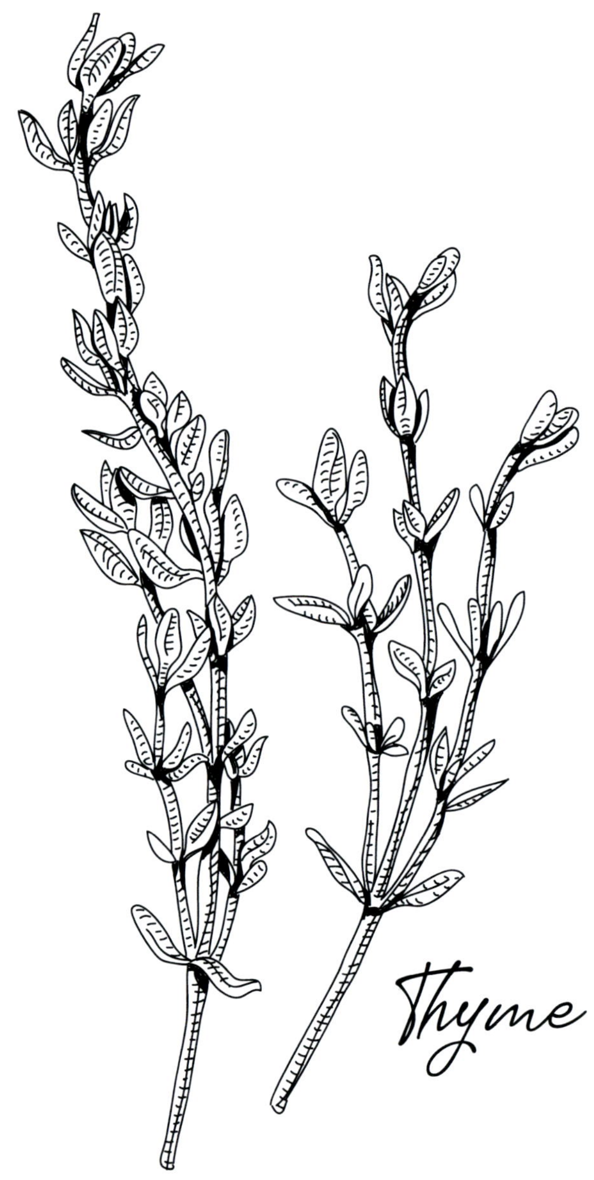

Thyme

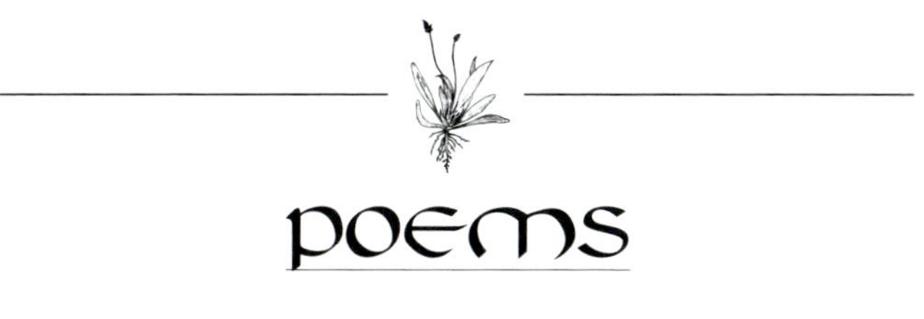

POEMS

ABOUT THE POEMS

All three of these poems are about my relationship with healing herbs and the world of nature. Like the stories, they came to me "out of the air" and as each one came, I memorized it.

WILLOWS AT IMBOLC came to me one Spring in the early 1980s, shortly after the February Cross-Quarter Day of Imbolc (Feast of Bridget or Candlemas). As I drove Purdon Road on the San Juan Ridge, day after day, year after year, I passed a beautiful Willow Bottom. Every year as January came to an end I watched closely as life came into the tips of the Willows until they were a vibrant yellow. Willows are the harbingers of Spring in our foothill habitat, and every year I watch them as they come out of dormancy and burn bright yellow until the magical moment when the new green growth springs forth in early February. But even in my New York childhood Willow was an infallible sign of spring. Every year in February my mother would come home bringing a couple branches of Pussy Willow to grace our apartment.

AUBADE came to me when I lived on Caney Fork in the Smoky Mountains of North Carolina. I was working on Tommy Beutell's Wolf Creek Christmas Tree Farm for $1 an hour. I was one of only two non-mountain people on the crew. One job was planting new fields on the nearly vertical slopes. We carried the long-rooted fir tree seedlings in a long cloth sack which dragged on the ground behind us. The task was to take a step, make a wedge shaped gash in the stiff soil with a mattock, jam a fir tree seedling into the gap and stamp it in. Then take another step and plant another seedling, all day long for ten or twelve hours.

As Christmas approached, we started cutting the trees from the mature fields and dragging them, two in each hand, down those steep slopes, piling them up to be taken by pick-up truck to the loading zone.

Once Christmas season arrived we worked by kerosene lantern light, often until after midnight, tossing fir trees up over the sides of stake bed trucks that would take them to the Christmas tree lots in the foothills and flat lands of North Carolina.

It was the physicality of tossing trees into the high-sided trucks that inspired this poem— the drops of icy water falling down my neck from each tree I lifted and tossed...the baffling places I would find fir needles the next day... the heady balsam perfume permeating my clothing and hair...the bloody scratches from the stiff, sharp branches.... All these physical experiences translated themselves into a visit from an invisible Fir Tree Spirit lover.

"Aubade" is an old term for a song of lovers' parting at dawn.

GIVING THANKS came to me one summer evening in the mid 1970s when I was drying herbs in my little cabin on Caney Fork. Jackson County got over 100 inches of rain every year, which made it very difficult to dry herbs quickly to the ideal state of "chip dry". ("Chip dry" means the leaf will snap like a crisp potato chip.) I had a rack from floor to ceiling with screen bottomed shelves. It stood right next to the wood burning stove in the living room. Thus the anomaly of burning "fat pine" in June. But such was the reality of the moment. "Fat pine" is the resin-rich heartwood of certain pine stumps. It burns very fast and very hot.

WILLOWS AT IMBOLC

Winter passes into Spring
a cool rain falls
and
      Willows
         burn
            bright
like tips of living flame

One more warm day
will see these slender withies
      burst
         and burn
with greener fire

— *Blind Shady, San Juan Ridge,*
California, 1983 in the days
leading up to Candlemas

AUBADE

I have a Fir Tree Spirit for a lover
I know him though I've never seen his face

Each morning when I wake—
      a memory of icy tears dropped on my breasts
      thighs, wrists scratched from his embrace

His pungent smell upon me

And balsam needles in my private place

— *Working on Tommy Beutell's Christmas Tree Farm,*
December 1972, Cullowhee, North Carolina

— *Published in Kyoi #2: A Journal of Back Country*
Writing, May, 1973

GIVING THANKS

A cricket singing on the door stop
fat pine burning in hot stove
mixed smell of elder blossoms drying—
      horsetail
      comfrey
      auger's yarrow
and pungent wormwood, feathery green

These herbs I dry on racks—
      stir
        turn
     and stir again until they snap
      chip dry
between my testing fingers

Then stored away in air-tight darkness
      they wait—
till some sharp winter need calls forth healing
      locked this night
in leaf and stem

So dreaming this June night
I sit
on dark porch rocking
breathing
deeply

— *Caney Fork, North Carolina, 1974*

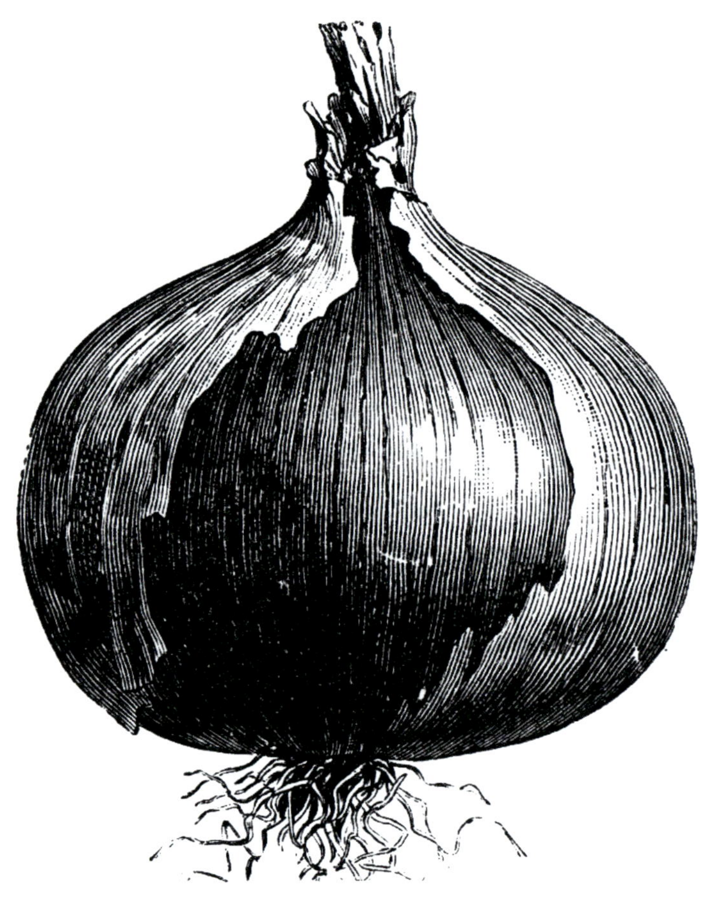

Onion

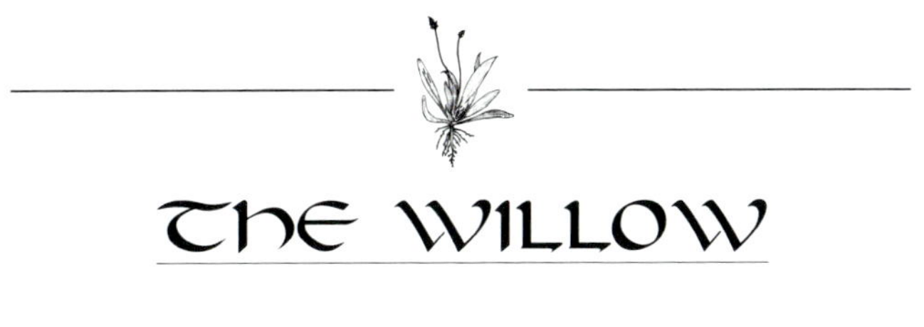

Che WILLOW

THE WILLOW IN STORY, SONG, AND EVERYDAY LIFE

The Willow is a very special plant. It is not only used for medicine, it is found in songs, tales, parables and mythology, plus it is useful for a number of applications in everyday life.

The Willow is famous in modern medicine because the salicins it contains led to the discovery of the drug we know as aspirin, which is now manufactured in laboratories rather than being extracted from the plant as an infusion.

One of the Celtic Tree Months is named for the Willow and the image of the Willow has been stitched into countless cross-stitch samplers of earlier centuries. It has always been, and remains, an important basket making material, as well as being used for building fences and other structures.

In the Celtic Tree Calendar, each of the thirteen lunar months is named for a tree—the one that is flowering or fruiting or otherwise notable at that time. The lunar calendar was our first calendar. Indeed, the word "month" comes from "moon". The Moon of the Willow is named "Saille".

In the more fluid lunar calendar, the Cross-Quarter Days (Seasonal Changes) and Quarter Days (Solstices and Equinoxes) are not locked onto the same day every year as they are in our fixed solar calendar introduced by Pope Gregory XIII in 1582. Rather, the Quarter and Cross-Quarter Days move back and forth between two adjacent months from year to year.

According to the Celtic Tree Calendar, the Cross-Quarter day of Beltane (May Day) can fall either in the Moon of Saille (Willow) or the Moon of Uath (Hawthorn). In olden days the May maidens in Britain used to carry Willow baskets filled with the ethereal white blossoms of the Hawthorn tree, also called the May tree.

Of all the trees, the Willow seems to occupy a special place in the hearts and minds of the people world-wide, because it is honored in songs, parables, stories and art. One example is the countless cross-stitch samplers of the 18th, 19th and early 20th centuries in which the Weeping Willow appears as a traditional mortuary motif.

THE WILLOW IN SONG

The Willow is found in many songs, usually associated with love and loss. These songs are from my own repertoire.

Oh bury me beneath that Willow
'Neath that weeping Willow tree
And when he comes he'll find me sleeping
Then perhaps he'll think of me
   Bury Me Beneath that Willow

Come all you young maidens,
  take warning from me
Never place your affections
  on a green Willow tree
For the leaves they will wither,
  and the roots they will die
And you'll all be forsaken
  and know not for why
   On Top of Old Smoky

Proud Maisrie stands at her faither's door
As straucht's a Willow wand
  The Gairdner's Chyld (Scottish)

The wind in the Willows
Crying like a solitary soul alone
  Round learned from my mother

And the Willow it shall weep,
And the Willow it shall whine
I wish I was in that young man's arms
That stole this heart of mine
  When I Was in My Prime

Ah bitter withy, ah bitter withy
And the Willow it doth smart
And the Willow shall be the very first tree
To perish at the heart
  The Bitter Withy
(the full text of *The Bitter Withy* is in the section on Songs)

On a tree by a river a little tom-tit
Sang "Willow, titwillow, titwillow"
And I said to him, "Dicky-bird, why do you sit
Singing 'Willow, titwillow, titwillow'"
"Is it weakness of intellect, birdie?" I cried
"Or a rather tough worm on your little insides?"
With a shake of his poor little head he replied
"Oh Willow, titwillow, titwillow"
  first verse from "Tit Willow" from "The Mikado" by Gilbert and Sullivan

And the blues song from the 1930s, "Willow Weep for Me", sung so beautifully by Billie Holiday, Sarah Vaughan, Nina Simone and others.

The only other trees I can think of being mentioned in folk ballads are the Oak and the Thorn in these two verses from "The Cruel Mother":

  She leaned her back against an Oak
    All alone and loney
  First it bent and then it broke
    Down by the greenwood sidey

  She leaned her back against a Thorn
    All alone and loney
  There she had two babies born
    Down by the greenwood sidey

(Don't you wish you knew what happened next?)

Add Ash to Oak and Thorn, and you have Oak, Ash and Thorn, the triumvirate of Celtic Wicca. Add Mistletoe to the Oak and you have Oak and Mistletoe, the primal pair Odin and Loki of Scandinavian mythology. Using heroic self-discipline, I am not going to digress into a discussion of Mistletoe.

THE WILLOW IN STORIES

The most famous literary reference I can think of must be the title of Kenneth Graeme's wonderful book *The Wind in the Willows* with its unforgettable characters Mole, Badger, Rat and Toad. And then there is the Whomping Willow in the Harry Potter tales.

The parable below was told to me by my mother when I was very young, probably for the reason all parables are told—to teach. In this case to teach me about two different ways of thinking and being. This is a paraphrase as I do not remember the story word for word as told to me.

The Oak and the Willow
Two trees stood in the meadow. A tall, proud and mighty Qak stood in the center and a slender, flexible Willow grew down on the edges where the meadow became moist bottom land. The Oak was proud in its strength and refused to bow or bend. The Willow made no such claim, being but a clump of slender, flexible withies. One night a terrible storm came and lashed the meadow all night with strong winds. In the morning, the mighty Oak, so proud that it refused to bend, was broken by the wind and lay splintered on the ground. The slender Willow was flexible and was willing to bend with the wind, so it was not harmed.

THE USEFUL WILLOW

The Medicinal Willow
One of the most well-known attributes of the Willow (*Salix* genus) is that the bark contains salicin, which is converted by the digestive processes into salicylic acid, a potent analgesic, anti-inflammatory and blood thinner. From this property of the Willow aspirin was "discovered". As is often the case when an herbal medicine is turned into a pharmaceutical, what is considered the "active ingredient" is isolated in the laboratory. This means that all the other bio-chemical constituents which potentize and *buffer* salicylic acid are now lacking. Herbal medicines are complex and have hundreds of constituents, all of which are active and needed to create the synergy that gives any herb its particular powers. When isolating a single "active ingredient", much is lost. That is why a single herb may be good for many conditions. What it is "good for" may depend on which part of the herb is used or how it is prepared. The truth is that herbs are complex and any given herb works in many ways, on many levels.

In the earlier section on *Herbal Compresses, Baths and Soaks,* I gave you the recipes for Willow Bark and Fucus hand and foot soaks. Alternating hand soaks of Willow bark and Fucus (Bladderwrack) for the arthritic CMC joint at the base of my thumb rid me of pain and averted my having to have surgery. An important thing to remember is that some people are allergic to salicins and may develop contact dermatitis from the Willow bark soak—I did when I failed to switch to Fucus soon enough. Wintergreen contains methyl salicylate, and should be avoided by people who are allergic to salicylic acid.

Sensitivity to salicylates is not uncommon. It can be upsetting to some stomachs as well.

Willow Baskets

The slender, flexible withies of the Willow are famous as basket making material. After the bark is peeled from the fresh withies, they are kept in a bucket of water to keep them flexible while you are weaving your basket. This is how I saw my mother do it.

Indigenous peoples of California prized Willow as a basketry material. Once peeled, it can be dyed with other plants and roots to create designs as the basket is woven. The People cultivated Willow by setting fire to the forest undergrowth right before they retired to their communal underground dwellings for the winter. These controlled burns kept the undergrowth down so that pre-European-contact forests were more like parks, easy to move through. They also made it possible for useful edible and medicinal plants that only grow up after a burn to be present when the People emerged in the spring. The burning back of old growth Willows allowed for a new crop of the slender, flexible, new withies to be immediately available for basketry, string and other

purposes. This annual burning of old-growth Willow also prevented the plant from growing into a tree whose wood was not useful because it would so easily "perish at the heart". Instead, an annual clump of useful, slender withies was assured.

Willow String

A single Willow withie can be split many times to make string. This Willow string is used in weaving, to bind the main weavers, especially when you are making a spiral, and for many other purposes as well. Coils of Willow bark string were once a common sight in the dwellings of Native Americans—for basketry and other uses. Willow string must be soaked to make it flexible for use. Once it dries and hardens, it is a supremely strong material.

Willow for the Gardener

If you stick a piece of freshly cut Willow in the ground it will instantly root, and you will have the beginnings of a Willow tree. This is because Willow contains rooting hormones.

The rooting compounds in Willow are indole butyric acid (IBA—found in commercial rooting products) and indole acetic acid (IAA). IAA is water soluble, so that is the ingredient that makes your homemade Willow rooting water so effective. In addition, Willow's salicins protect the baby roots of your starts from fungi.

Harvest two young Willow shoots, as long as your arm and no thicker than a pencil, remove the leaves, and snip the slender withies into 1" pieces. Put the pieces in a mason jar, pour in boiling water, cover and let steep for 24 hours, then strain. You can use your Willow brew to water in newly planted seedlings, or dilute it by half and use it for soaking your ready-to-plant seedlings or fresh cuttings in a jar before planting them. My mother used to snip a bunch of fresh Willow pieces and put them in the jar with the Rose cuttings she wanted to root.

Your Willow water can be stored in the fridge for two months, but be sure to let it return to room temperature before using it. Cold water will shock your seedlings.

Willow Fences

Fences made of Willow were once common in many European countries and among Native American tribes. They can be found wherever Willow grows, or is accessible, and I suspect Willow fences are still used in many places. They are easy and effective. You can find instructions online for several different methods for making Willow fences, and you can even buy pre-made rolls of Willow and wire fencing on Amazon!

Willow, when cut fresh and stuck immediately into the earth, will live, put out roots and continue to grow. When done right, you end up with a beautiful living Willow fence.

In 1917, the anthropologist Gilbert L. Wilson was smart enough to talk to Buffalo Bird Woman, and subsequently gave a meticulous description of this Hidatsa master gardener's practices in the book *Buffalo Bird Woman's Garden*, re-published by the Minnesota Historical Society Press in 1987. The following is a quotation from this wonderful book describing the way the Hidatsa made Willow fences.

> *Post holes were made by driving a sharp stake into the ground with an ax; the stake was withdrawn, and into the hole left by it, a diamond Willow was thrust for a post; on this Willow were left all the upper branches with the leaves. A rail was run from the post to its next neighbor, at the height of a woman's shoulder, and stayed in place by bending over the leafy top of the Willow post, and drawing it around the rail, then twisting it down and around the body of the post in a spiral manner. If the leafy top of the post was long enough, and slender enough, it might, after being wrapped spirally about the post, be even drawn out and woven into the fence.*
>
> *Below the top rail at a convenient distance, there ran a second rail, bound to the post with bark. [this would be the Willow string I described earlier]. Besides these rails, branches and twigs, and as I have said, the tops of the posts themselves, were interwoven into the fence to make it as dense as possible.*
>
> *The posts of the fence stood about two and a half feet apart, making, with the rails and the interwoven twigs, a barrier so dense that even a dog could not push through it.*
>
> *There was an opening left to enter the garden, closed by a kind of stile-bars of small poles thrust right and left between the posts; against these bars were leaned one or two bull berry bushes [Shepardia argentea], which were removed when the owner wanted to enter."*

A fence so dense even a dog could not force its way through would have been a very effective barrier to keep out all kind of critters.

The Willow-Framed Sweat Lodge

Although sweat bathing as a secular practice is found world-wide, from the Finnish sauna to the Turkish hammam, the Native American Sweat Lodge is a sacred place, a place of healing and prayer, a place of purification and of vision. As far as I know, the Sweat is ubiquitous in Native American cultures.

If you wish to learn more about the Native American Sweat Lodge, I recommend *The Native American Sweat Lodge: History and Legends* by Joseph Bruchac (The Crossing Press, 1933). Naturally, the materials from which the Sweat Lodge was built depended on the habitat and the materials available there.

My experience is with the Willow-framed Sweat Lodge. For fifteen years I drove two or three times a year from Grass Valley down Highway 395 (one of the two most beautiful drives in California) to Big Pine in Owens Valley, just below Bishop, in order to sweat with Raymond Stone, a Paiute healer famous among many other Native American healers, doctors and shamans.

A Sweat Lodge may be a small, temporary affair, big enough for one person, or a large, semi-permanent structure built to hold many people. Raymond's Sweat Lodge could hold twelve of us packed shoulder to shoulder.

To build a Sweat Lodge, first draw a circle on the ground using a peg and a string. The string should be the diameter of the circle you wish to create. This will give you the circumference of the Lodge. Now dig twelve deep, inward slanting holes around this circle which will hold the butts of the twelve big, strong, flexible white Willow saplings from which the framework is built. The inward slanting holes keep the butts of the structural Willow saplings from pulling out of the ground. The framework starts with these Willow poles which are bent over and lashed together at the top, forming hoops with the biggest hoop at the center. More Willow poles are woven horizontally into the twelve vertical poles, with the stoutest at the bottom and the finest at the top.

Before the cover goes on, the pit for the hot rocks is dug slightly to the front of the center of the Lodge, and the earth taken from the pit is used to construct a mound directly in front of the entrance. A buffalo skull is placed on this mound. A short distance from the mound is the fire pit in which the Sweat rocks are heated. Only volcanic rocks of a certain kind can be used—ordinary rocks shatter dangerously.

The covering of the Sweat Lodge is made up of layers—first came heavy, water-proofed canvas tarps, then blankets and quilts, then more canvas tarps, all lashed down securely by strong ropes. From a short distance, the Lodge looked like a giant turtle.

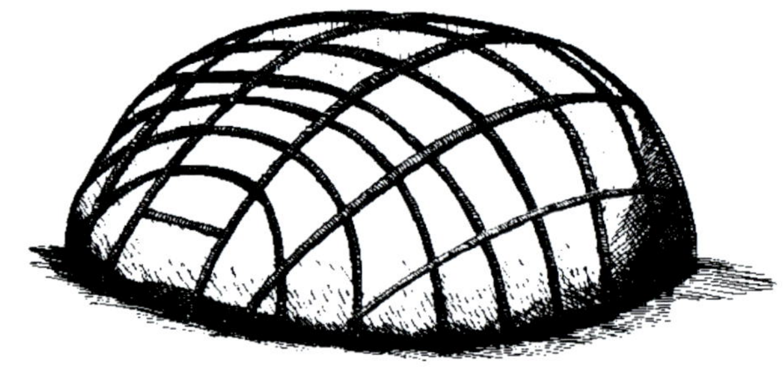

The Lodge is always constructed with a small opening on the east side for entering and exiting. It is covered with a flap during the Sweat. Some Lodges have an opening on the west side as well. In California, tules (large bulrushes found only in certain marshy areas of California) line the periphery of the inside of the Lodge, and it is on these tules that you sit.

If you ever have the opportunity to attend a Sweat Lodge, you will be grateful if you find yourself with one of the stout structural Willows supporting your back. And when you look up you will often see strings of tobacco ties (Strings of small cloth bundles, each containing a generous pinch of tobacco) woven into the structural Willows. Raymond tucked his eagle wing fan and other ceremonial objects into the handy Willow framework.

If you wish to read another description of the construction of the Sweat Lodge using Willow, see if you can find Reginald and Gladys Laubin's book, *The Indian Tipi: It's History, Construction and Use*, originally published by the University of Oklahoma Press. There is a whole chapter dedicated to the construction of a Willow-Framed Sweat Lodge. The Laubins spent time with the Indian Peoples of the Plains and Prairies—the Sioux, the Crow, the Arapahoe, the Cheyenne, and probably many more. Their description is remarkably like the way Raymond's Sweat Lodge was built and conducted.

You can find a more detailed description of the Sweat Lodge and my Pipe Fast and other details about Raymond's Sweat Lodge in the chapter "Marina's Story: The Rest of My Life" IN: *Going Up the Country: Adventures in Blues Fieldwork in the 1960s*, published by the University Press of Mississippi, Fall 2022.

<u>Willow for Wattle and Daub Construction</u>
In the olden days, one of the easiest, cheapest and sturdiest ways to build a house or other kind of structure was the wattle and daub method. Wattle and daub (which might also be called "sticks and mud") construction can be found all over the world—from simple round huts in Africa to multi-story "Tudor style" buildings in Europe, some of which have wattle and daub walls which are at least 700 years old. So it is definitely a durable method of building. Historically, it is one of the most common wall infill techniques for timber framed houses.

Although any kind of wood can be used, wattle and daub construction most often uses the withies from pollarded trees, and withies from flexible plants like Willow and Hazel. The Willow is exceptionally well suited for making the woven lattice framework which makes up the "wattle" part of the construction. The "daub" is the local clayey subsoil, often mixed with animal dung and other plant material—just as straw is needed to make bricks. I imagine that with a layer of daub on the outside of the woven wattle, and a layer of daub on the inside, which would probably be whitewashed or plastered, a wattle and daub building would be naturally well insulated.

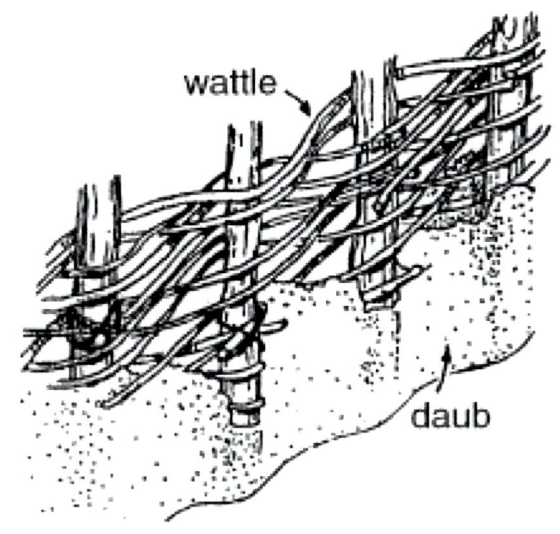

Check out this article which is a nice introduction to wattle and daub building:
https://www.lowimpact.org/lowimpact-topic/wattle-daub/

I had to keep myself from going down this very fascinating wattle-and-daub rabbit-hole. Simply search "wattle and daub Pinterest" to see many pages devoted to this building technique. Here is a handful of my favorite pages:

- **https://www.pinterest.com/sissybeam/wattle-and-daub/**
Lots of Tudor, one primitive round, shows building of a low wattle and daub wall.

- **https://za.pinterest.com/gardiner-megan2/wattle-and-daub-walls/**
Shows a simple corner technique, focus on wall techniques.

- **https://www.pinterest.com/kmcranch/wattle-and-daub/**
Lots of fences and good illustration of construction methods.

- **https://www.pinterest.com/brendal-hicks77/wattle-daub/**
Shows step by step building of a small shed.

- **https://www.pinterest.com/search/pins/?q=wattle%20and%20daub&rs-=typed&term_meta%5b%5d=wa-ttle%20and%20daub%7Ctyped**
This page has many, many pictures of all kinds of wattle and daub buildings.

Suffice it to say, Willow is a truly flexible (pun intended) building material, well suited for framing a Sweat Lodge, making impenetrable fences, and creating wattle and daub architecture. Wattle and daub is again becoming popular as a low cost, low-impact, ecologically intelligent method of building.

Willow is but one plant that has multiple uses. I hope my *Simpler's Garland* has given you a little taste for the beauty and utility of a some of our plant friends. And there are so many, many more for which I did not have space. And there are even more of which I do not yet know. One never stops learning.

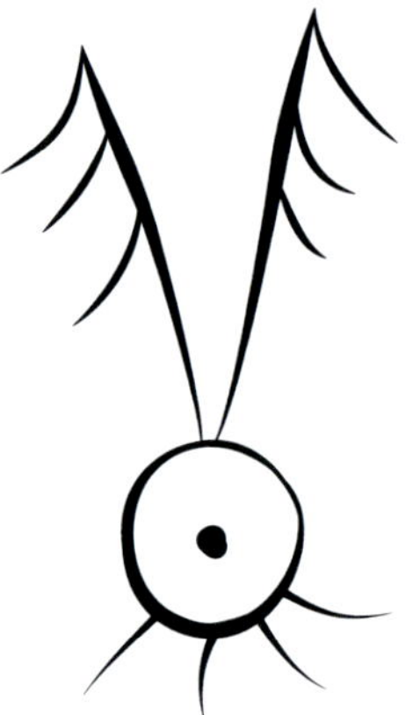

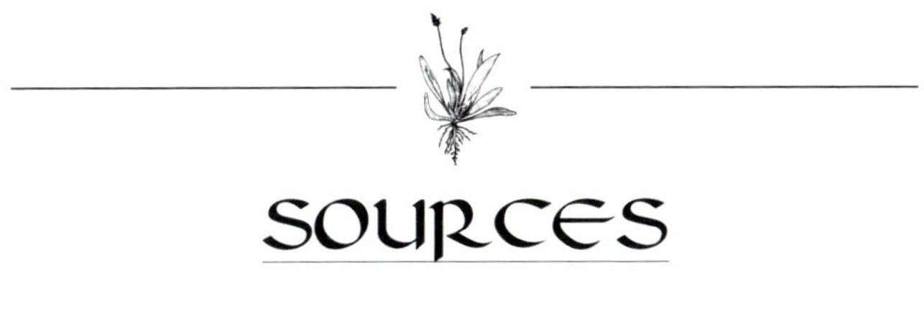

SOURCES

MEDICINE FLOWER HEALING HERBAL SALVES
Linda Gordon
541-366-2053 (landline)
530-802-1632 (cell)
medicine.flower72@gmail.com

SACRED PAW PUBLICATIONS
The writings of Marina Bokelman
Jill Kelly

Sacredpaw1992@gmail.com

Cheryl Thurber, Literary Agent/Executor
443-630-0672
cthurb@yahoo.com
litery.ex@gmail.com

ALL MY RELATIONS

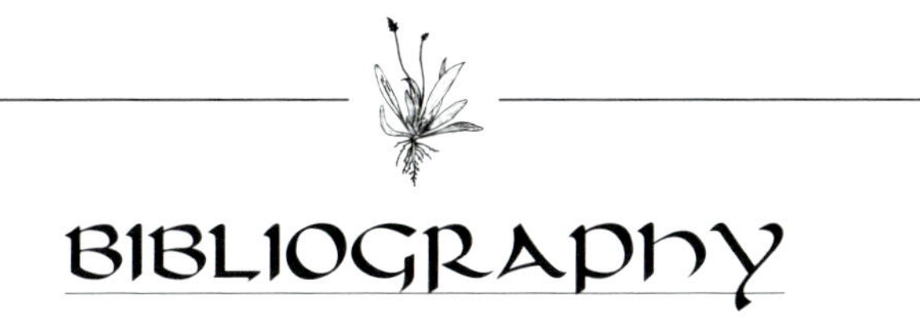

BIBLIOGRAPHY

SACRED PAW PRESS: The Writtings of Marina Bokelman

My Paw Is Sacred; All Things Are Sacred

Tobaccos I Have Grown and Loved, 2021
Cover art by Cat Raymond, color photographs, acid free paper.

In this unique chapbook Marina talks about her years growing Native American species of *Nicotiana* (Tobacco). She describes five of her favorites, and gives detailed instructions for germinating tobacco from seed, transplanting it into the garden, growing for harvesting of leaf and viable seeds. She describes her simple methods for curing tobacco on baskets, discusses pollinators and pests, and reports scientific findings on the biological intelligence of *Nicotiana attenuata*. She touches on issues of tobacco addiction and withdrawal, and the use of tobacco as an entheogen.

A Simpler's Garland: The Gentle Art of Poulticing and Other Herbal Writings of Marina Bokelman, 2021
Black and white botanical illustrations.

Based on a revised and enlarged version of her article on poulticing published in *Mothering Magazine*, this book also contains Marina's *Herb Talk* articles in Nevada City's *The Independent* newspaper. She lists useful poulticing herbs: raw green herbs, roots, garlic, cucurbits, plus dried and powdered herbs. She describes her experiences with simple and compound poultices, and with herbal baths and soaks. She gives detailed instructions for her own method of making herbal salves. This interesting and valuable book also contains songs, poems and tales based on herbal lore, and a chapter on The Useful Willow.

The Tale of the Shirt: How Dale Pendell's Power Shirt Came to Be, 2021
Thirty-five stunning color photographs by Hank Meals, black and white and color photographs, and a color reproduction from Dale's silk-screened masterpiece: *The Gold Dust Wilderness*.

Marina gives an account of her friendship with Dale Pendell—poet, artist, writer, ethnobotanist, philosopher—and describes the two pieces of embroidery she made for him: a Huichol inspired cross-stitched Medicine Pouch, and what Dale called his "Power Shirt". She describes the free-form embroidery techniques she used to create the Shirt as a model of the Cosmos, and how she represented the California Native American view of the Creation of the Universe through Chumash and Inyo inspired pictographs and petroglyphs. She speaks of embroidery as a form of Practice, and tells the California Native creation myths represented by the various groupings of glyphs on the Shirt.

Contact Sacred Paw Press:
Jill Kelly
Sacredpaw1992@gmail.com

<u>OTHER PUBLICATIONS OF MARINA BOKELMAN</u>

<u>UNIVERSITY PRESS OF MISSISSIPPI</u>

Marina Bokelman and David Evans
<u>Going Up the Country:</u>
<u>Adventures in Blues Fieldwork in the 1960s</u>.
    The story of two young white graduate students from UCLA and their adventures in Mississippi and Louisiana doing blues field work in the 1960s. Their story is told through the fieldnotes of Bokelman and Evans written at the time, and edited later by Bokelman, and by over 100 vintage photographs taken by Marina Bokelman while in the field. The book also contains retrospective writings by Bokelman and Evans, and scholarly essays about bluesmen and their careers written by Evans. Bibliography; Archival Resources. Projected publication, late Fall, 2022.

<u>Order through your local bookstore or contact UPM</u>:
— ***Direct order number:***
   1-800-737-7788
— ***Sandy Alexander, Orders Director***
   601-432-6704
   <u>salexander@ihl.state.ms.us</u>

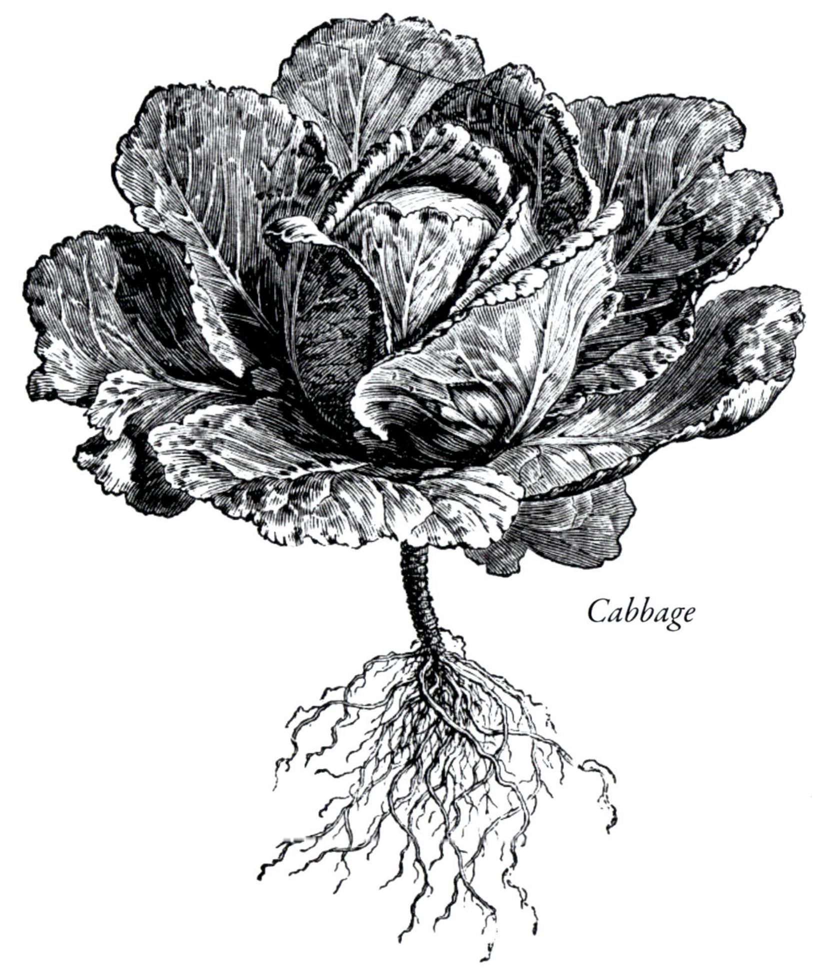

Cabbage

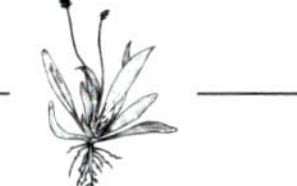

ARCHIVAL RESOURCES

*"**Ethnomusicology Archive: D. K. Wilgus Collection**", **UCLA Library, Digital Collections**,* Search under *David Evans* or *Marina Bokelman* or name of interviewee. Field recordings and interviews by both collectors, 1965-1968.
https://digital2.library.ucla.edu/

*"**The Marina Bokelman Collection**"* at **The Blues Archive, University of Mississippi, Archives and Special Collections, John Davis William Library**. Internet search under "Marina Bokelman Finding Aid Ole Miss" for complete details. Recordings of Canned Heat in rehearsal and performance, interviews with each band member, transcriptions of interviews, 8mm film from an uncompleted documentary film, negatives of photographs, contact sheets and more.
Collection No.: MUM00584. Greg Johnson, Archivist, (662) 915-71408, gj1@olemiss.edu

*"**The Marina Bokelman Collection**"* at **The Southern Folklife Collection, Louis Round Wilson Library, Special Collections, University of North Carolina, Chapel Hill,** Original negatives, contact sheets and field notes documenting 1966-1968 fieldwork in Mississippi, Louisiana and California; the original hand written field notes of Marina Bokelman; M.A. thesis: "The Coon Can Game: A Blues Ballad Tradition"; books written by Marina Bokelman; media containing Marina's photographs; cross-stitch sampler commissioned by Bill Givens of Origin Jazz Library Records for the cover of OJL-21; more.
Collection No.:70035. *Steve Weiss, Curator, (919) 962-7105 smweiss@email.unc.edu*

*"**The Marina Bokelman Collection**"* at **The Searls Historical Library, Archive of the Nevada County Historical Society, Nevada City, CA.** Sponsored by a grant from the California Arts Council, the collection documents the social and cultural life of the San Juan Ridge, 1982-1985: recordings of storytelling and musical events at the North Columbia Schoolhouse Cultural Center and of "Old Timers' Night" and other events at the Fire Hall; oral histories of old timers; recordings of *Folk Plus,* an educational folk music program produced by Marina for KVMR. Also: recordings of radio interviews with and studio recordings of Marina Bokelman, folksinger/guitarist and *a cappella* ballad singer; Marina's *Herb Talk* articles in *The Independent* newspaper and more. **Digital catalog search under: Marina Bokelman, San Juan Ridge Research, California Arts Council Grant, San Juan Ridge.**
Director, Pat Chesnut, (530) 265-5910 pchesnut@hughes.net

IN: *"The Dale Pendell Papers"*, <u>**Special Collections, Shields Library University of California, Davis;**</u> *The Tale of the Shirt: How Dale Pendell's Power Shirt Came to Be" a book by Marina Bokelman with many color photographs by Hank Meals*; the original Medicine Shirt and Medicine Pouch embroidered by Marina Bokelman; the correspondence of Dale Pendell and Marina Bokelman.
Collection No: D-710. *Head Archivist, Kevin Miller, (530) 7521621 <u>kcmiller@ucdavis.edu</u> or <u>SpecColl@ucdavis.edu</u>*

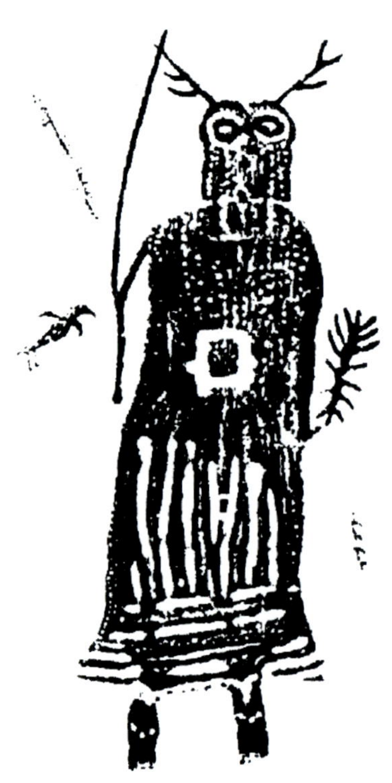

BY THIS MERIT
MAY ALL BEINGS BENEFIT